KW-051-212

DEPARTMENT OF COMMUNITY MEDICINE

Epidemiology of Musculoskeletal Disorders

Monographs in Epidemiology and Biostatistics
edited by Abraham M. Lilienfeld

Monographs in Epidemiology and Biostatistics
Volume 3

Epidemiology of Musculoskeletal Disorders

by
Jennifer L. Kelsey

YALE UNIVERSITY SCHOOL OF MEDICINE
DEPARTMENT OF EPIDEMIOLOGY AND PUBLIC HEALTH

New York   Oxford
OXFORD UNIVERSITY PRESS
1982

Copyright © 1982 by Oxford University Press, Inc.

Library of Congress Cataloging in Publication Data

Kelsey, Jennifer L.
  Epidemiology of musculoskeletal disorders.

  (Monographs in epidemiology and biostatistics ; v. 3)
  Bibliography: p.
  Includes index.
  1. Musculoskeletal system—Diseases.   2. Musculoskeletal
system—Abnormalities.   3. Epidemiology.   I. Title.
II. Series. [DNLM: 1. Muscular diseases—Occurrence.
2. Bone diseases—Occurrence. WE 140 K295e]
RA645.M85K44   614.5′97   82–3511
ISBN 0–19–503117–2

Printing (last digit): 9 8 7 6 5 4 3 2 1

Printed in the United States of America

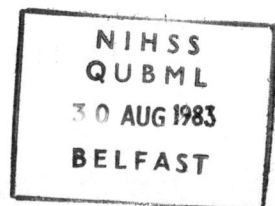

NIHSS
QUBML
3 0 AUG 1983
BELFAST

Preface

Musculoskeletal disorders are a major public health problem in most parts of the world, yet relatively few studies have been undertaken of the epidemiology of most of these conditions. Furthermore, there have been few review articles written on epidemiologic aspects of individual disorders, let alone of all the major musculoskeletal conditions.

This book brings together and critically analyzes the relevant literature on the epidemiology of the major musculoskeletal disorders. Although the text was written by an epidemiologist primarily for epidemiologists and other public health practitioners, many of whom have little knowledge of the disease processes involved, it is hoped that orthopedists, rheumatologists, and other physicians will skip over the simplified descriptions of the diseases and find the epidemiologic material instructive and enlightening.

There is a certain unevenness in the quantity and quality of the material presented on the different diseases. In part, this may reflect the author's more extensive experience in some areas than in others and to her greater depth of knowledge of some diseases than others. However, there is also tremendous variation in the amount of information available on the epidemiology of the various diseases, and while a few diseases have been studied fairly extensively, no epidemiologic studies have been undertaken of many of them. Accordingly, throughout the book many preliminary findings are presented that are in need of further study.

It is hoped that readers will note the many gaps in the understanding of the epidemiology of these diseases and will recognize the areas in which further study is needed. One important service this book could perform would be as an impetus for other investigators to undertake their own studies to enhance our understanding of the epidemiology of musculo-skeletal disorders. In light of the high frequency of these conditions in the population, any new information that could be used to prevent their occurrence or to reduce their impact would certainly be of benefit to society.

New Haven   J. L. K.
October 1981

Acknowledgments

This book would not have been possible without the substantial, generous, and willing help of several people. First, thanks go to Dr. Abraham M. Lilienfeld for initiating and encouraging this series of books, and for his extremely helpful comments on the manuscript. Troy Holbrook contributed considerably to the literature review for the chapter on arthritic disorders, Sue Egerter to the chapter on congenital malformations, and Gretchen Dieck and Nancy Kreiger to various sections of the book. Special thanks for typing go to Ellen Bedard and Barbara Hoxsie and for supervision and technical editing to Penny Githens; these three individuals worked long hours with great cheerfulness and efficiency. Also contributing in various ways were Coleen Boyle, Priscilla Canny, Patricia Caplan, Linda Cunningham, Kathleen Derr, Nancy Hildreth, Marika Iwane, Cindy Jajich, and Peter Kalamarides. The support of Beryl Gillette, Eppie and Gwen Kelsey, Sharon Ort, and Virginia Richards throughout the preparation of the book has been of tremendous help. Phillip Parker of Oxford University Press helped considerably in the preparation of the final manuscript. In fact, it would be difficult to assembly a more helpful group than all those mentioned above.

Contents

Epidemiology of Musculoskeletal Disorders

1 Introduction

Disorders of the musculoskeletal system are among the most common afflictions of the human race. They affect all age groups and are associated with a great deal of disability, impairment, and handicap. Musculoskeletal disorders encompass a variety of conditions, ranging in severity from relatively minor aches and pains such as mild cases of "dog-walker's elbow (6)" to chronic disabling diseases such as rheumatoid arthritis. Although musculoskeletal conditions are occasionally fatal, their main impact is on quality of life and on economic productivity.

This preliminary chapter introduces the book in two ways: (a) an overview is given of the impact that musculoskeletal disorders have as a group; a more comprehensive review of this material is available elsewhere (4); (b) the limitations of the material presented in subsequent chapters are discussed, as it seems important for the reader to realize at the outset how little is known of the epidemiology of many musculoskeletal diseases and to understand that much of the material to be presented should be regarded as preliminary leads for further investigation.

MAGNITUDE OF THE PROBLEM

According to the Health Interview Survey of the U.S. National Health Survey, which divides health problems into acute and chronic conditions, each year in the United States there are about 14.5 episodes per 100 people of injuries or acute diseases of the musculoskeletal system of sufficient severity to warrant medical care or restriction of activity (16). Among all

3

Table 1-1 Estimated Numbers of Individuals Who Reported Selected Impairments in Past Year, Health Interview Survey: United States, 1971

Type of impairment	Estimated number of individuals	
Musculoskeletal impairments	18,879,000	
(except paralysis or amputation)		
Back or spine		8,018,000
Lower extremity or hip		7,387,000
Upper extremity or shoulder		2,440,000
Other or multiple		1,034,000
Hearing impairments	14,491,000	
Visual impairments	9,596,000	
Speech defects	1,934,000	
Paralysis, complete or partial	1,392,000	
Absence of entire finger(s) or toe(s) only	858,000	
Absence of major extremities	274,000	

Source: National Center for Health Statistics, Health Interview Survey (9).

categories of acute conditions, musculoskeletal disorders rank second in frequency after acute respiratory conditions.

Of even greater importance, however, is the chronicity of many musculoskeletal disorders. Table 1-1 presents the estimated number of individuals who reported various impairments in the Health Interview Survey of 1971, an impairment being defined as a chronic or permanent defect representing a decrease or loss of ability to perform various functions. It may be seen that musculoskeletal conditions were the most common type of impairment among those considered (9), affecting about 10 percent of the population. In fact, musculoskeletal conditions were the most frequently reported impairment among both males and females in each of the three age groups into which the population was divided (less than 45 years of age, 45 to 64 years, 65 years and older). Table 1-1 also shows that the back or spine is the part of the musculoskeletal system most frequently affected, followed by the lower extremity or hip, and the upper extremity or shoulder.

Figure 1-1 indicates that over 10 million people in the United States have their activity limited by musculoskeletal diseases, a number greater than that for any other disease category (22). In this graph, fractures, dislocations, sprains, and strains are counted in the "accidents, poisonings, and violence" category, so that the actual reported number of people with their activity limited by musculoskeletal disorders is slightly higher

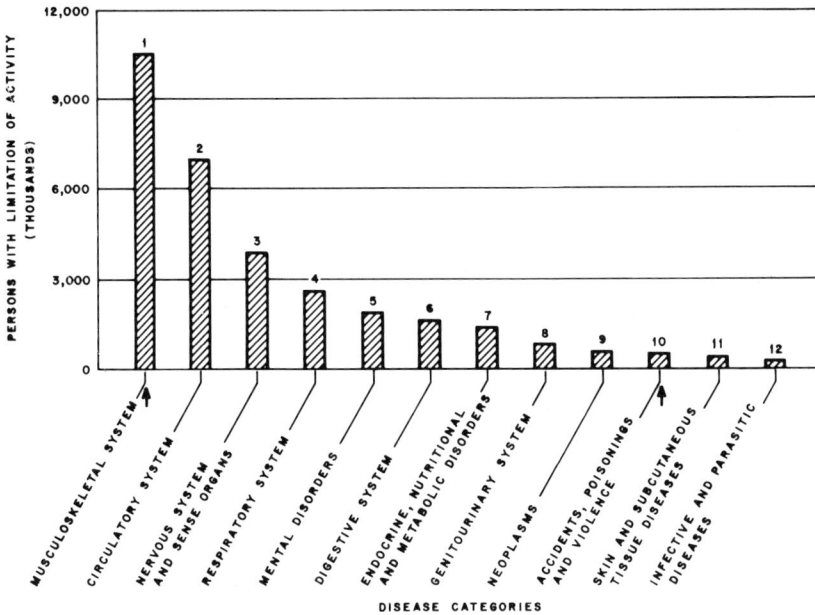

Figure 1-1   Estimated number of persons in United States in 1971 with limitation of activity attributable to specific conditions.

Source: From Life and Death and Medicine, by Kerr L. White. Copyright © 1973 by Scientific American, Inc. All rights reserved.

than that indicated in the figure. Figure 1-2 shows that heart disease ranks first in the percentage of persons with a chronic condition whose activity is limited because of the condition, followed by arthritis and rheumatism, impairments of the lower extremities and hips, and impairments of the back and spine. When mobility limitation is considered (Figure 1-3), arthritis and rheumatism ranks first and impairments of the lower extremities and hips second. Almost one-quarter of persons who report having arthritis and rheumatism have their mobility limited because of it.

Musculoskeletal disorders are most frequent among the elderly, among whom the course may be severe. A study in England (19) revealed that many of the elderly affected with musculoskeletal disorders lived alone; half of them had difficulties imposed by stairs within or at the entrance to their home, and one-third said they would not even be able to attract attention in an emergency. Twenty percent were dependent on others for such ordinarily routine tasks as taking a bath, doing housework, cutting

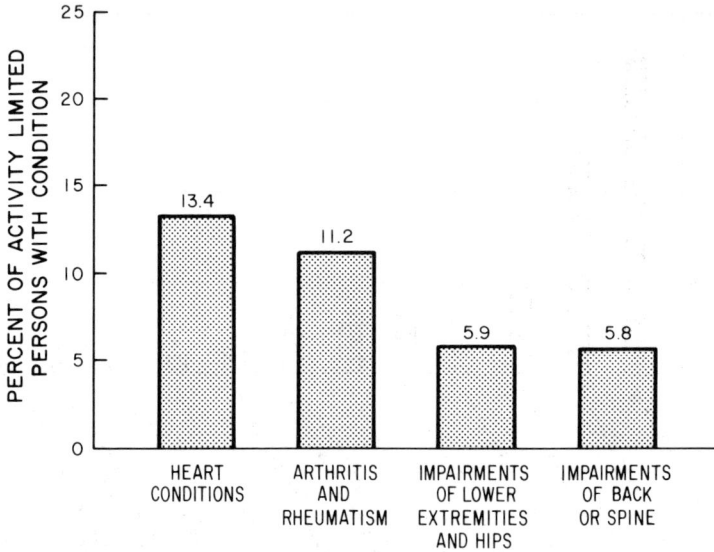

Figure 1-2 Percentage of persons with activity limitation who reported selected chronic conditions as the main cause of their limitation.

Source: National Center for Health Statistics (8).

Figure 1-3 Percentage of persons with mobility limitation who reported selected chronic conditions as the main cause of their limitation.

Source: National Center for Health Statistics (8).

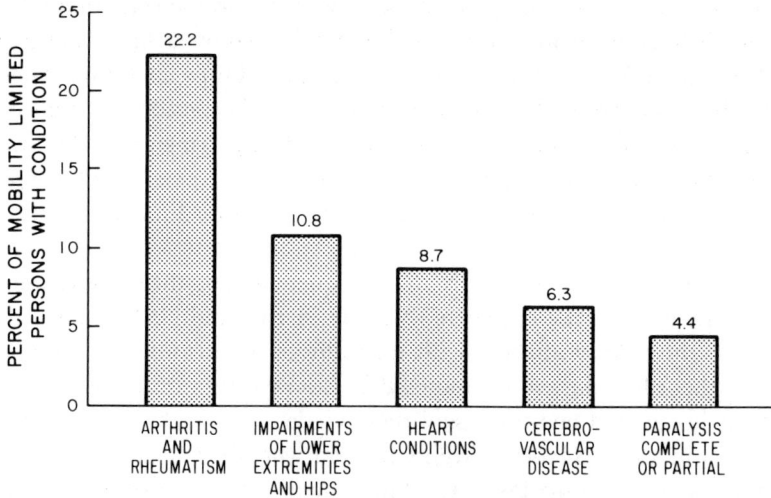

toenails, or getting out of the house. Another indicator of the large impact on the elderly is the cost to Medicare in the United States, as about 20 percent of Medicare hospitalization costs are for musculoskeletal conditions. Among the musculoskeletal conditions, hip fracture is the most frequent and by far the most costly reason for hospitalization in the age group 65 years and older. Osteoarthrosis and fractures of other sites are also common and costly (18,21).

Musculoskeletal disorders have a large impact on people in their productive working years. A study of people of ages 18 to 64 years showed that musculoskeletal conditions are the leading cause of disability (3). In this age group, about 2 percent of the population is disabled from arthritis and rheumatism and about 2 percent from impairments of the back and spine. About one-third of those disabled with arthritis and rheumatism and over one-fifth of those disabled with impairments of the back and spine were classified as being severely disabled. Data from the U.S. National Health Survey (15) indicate that the average worker loses 5.2 days from work in a year because of illnesses and injuries, and it is estimated that 1.9 of these days are attributable to musculoskeletal conditions (4,14). Impairments of the back and spine and arthritis and rheumatism account for the greatest amount of time lost from work (7). In 1976, it was reported that a reduction of one day per year in the average annual absenteeism rate among the labor force of the United States would increase the gross national product (GNP) by $10,000 million. Accordingly, the GNP would have increased by $19,000 million had musculoskeletal disorders been prevented. Considering the extent of inflation since 1976, this estimate would undoubtedly be higher now. According to data from the U.S. Social Security Administration, musculoskeletal conditions rank second to diseases of the circulatory system as a cause of disability in workers; 17 percent of workers given disability allowances receive them because of musculoskeletal diseases. Table 1-2 shows that osteoarthrosis ranks second, displaced intervertebral discs third, and rheumatoid arthritis seventh among conditions for which worker disability allowances are granted (20).

Musculoskeletal disorders result in about 55 million visits to office-based physicians per year, a figure exceeded only by diseases of the respiratory system (82 million visits per year) (17). About 8.4 percent of hospitalizations (excluding deliveries) in short-stay hospitals in the United States are for musculoskeletal disorders (10), placing them fourth in frequency among males and sixth among females (11). On the average, patients with musculoskeletal disorders stay in the hospital 5 to 7 days,

Table 1-2 Most Frequent Conditions for Which Worker Disability Allowances Were Granted by the Social Security System by Sex, United States, 1973

Condition	Total	Males	Females
Chronic ischemic heart disease	104,483	82,099	22,384
Osteoarthrosis	29,464	18,721	10,743
Displacement of intervertebral disc	20,084	14,712	5,372
Emphysema	17,837	15,401	2,436
Schizophrenia	17,701	12,467	5,234
Diabetes mellitus	13,116	8,391	4,725
Rheumatoid arthritis	11,347	5,776	5,571

Source: Social Security Disability Applicant Statistics, 1973 (20).

a longer period of time than for most other diseases. Orthopedic operations are third in frequency among surgical procedures in short-stay hospitals in the United States; among all operations, about 13 percent are estimated to be orthopedic (12).

Musculoskeletal disorders are not among the most important causes of death. When associated with mortality, it is usually in the category of accidents, which are the fourth-leading cause of death in all ages and the leading cause of death from ages 1 to 34 years (13).

Finally, the estimated total economic cost to the United States of musculoskeletal conditions is second only to that of diseases of the circulatory system (2,4). Indirect costs from lost earnings and services represent a particularly high proportion of the total cost, since many people are affected during their most productive years.

LIMITATIONS OF EPIDEMIOLOGIC DATA

Despite the importance of musculoskeletal disorders both to society and to the many individuals affected, subsequent chapters indicate how little is known of the epidemiology of many of these diseases. Epidemiologists have generally tended to focus on disorders associated with high mortality rates, such as cardiovascular diseases and cancers, rather than on diseases that primarily affect the quality of life. It is probably in part for this reason, and in part because of the relatively gradual onset and difficulty of diagnosis of some of the major musculoskeletal disorders, that so much remains to be learned of the epidemiology of these conditions.

Spina bifida cystica actually has been the subject of many epidemiologic studies, probably because this condition is sufficiently severe to be identified through hospital records, death certificates, or birth certificates. Other conditions, such as hip fracture (often used as an indicator of osteoporosis) and slipped epiphysis, which generally require hospitalization for treatment, have also been the subject of some epidemiologic study. However, the vast majority of musculoskeletal disorders are usually not fatal, are not necessarily seen in hospitals, have a gradual onset, and in many instances may not even come to medical attention. Accordingly, much of what is known about the epidemiology of these diseases has been limited to findings from reports of series of cases from individual physicians and hospitals. Not only are such series unrepresentative of cases from the general population, but the numbers studied are often small, and comparison groups are frequently not used. Many of the findings from such studies can be considered no more than clinical impressions that should be subject to further investigation. Even if all cases coming to medical attention within a defined geographic area are included in a study, the factors that bring persons with a given condition to medical attention often cannot be separated from factors that may be related to disease etiology. Thus, community surveys are necessary to learn about the epidemiology of many of these conditions.

Some population-based surveys have in fact been conducted, particularly for the arthritic disorders. However, diagnostic criteria for some of these diseases have been established only recently, little evaluation of the criteria has been undertaken, and the criteria are not always used uniformly. For diseases with no standard diagnostic criteria, geographical and temporal comparisons have very little meaning. An analogous situation exists for diseases that constitute one end of a continuous distribution, such as osteoporosis, scoliosis, and kyphosis. To define cases of these diseases, a more or less arbitrary cutoff point of what is disease and what is normal must be established, but unfortunately different investigators have chosen different cutoff points. It is also sometimes difficult to differentiate such diseases as osteoporosis, degenerative disc disease, and osteoarthrosis from the normal aging process.

Many musculoskeletal diseases have been divided into subcategories; for example, the three major types of clubfoot are talipes equinovarus, metatarsus varus, and talipes calcaneovalgus. Some studies have been limited to talipes equinovarus, others have included all three types, and some have not even indicated which types are included. In studies of certain other conditions, such as flat foot and limb reduction deformities, most investigators have used their own individual systems of subcategorization. "Unfortunately ... some authors would sooner use somebody else's toothbrush than his terminology (5)." Epidemiologic studies of back pain do not generally consider the many different causative disease processes; to a certain extent this is understandable since at present even the most sophisticated diagnostic procedures cannot determine the specific lesion responsible for the pain in most cases. However, much information is lost when diseases with differing etiologies are considered as a single disorder.

These are some of the major general problems that have limited current knowledge of the epidemiology of many of the musculoskeletal diseases. Problems peculiar to individual diseases or groups of diseases will be mentioned in the appropriate context. This brief overview of these limitations is not meant as a criticism of work that has already been done in the epidemiology of musculoskeletal disorders. Instead, these problems are presented at the outset so that the reader will exercise appropriate caution in interpreting the material to be described in subsequent chapters. Perhaps most important, readers should realize that epidemiologic knowledge of many disorders of the musculoskeletal system is in its infancy, and it is hoped that some readers will be encouraged to undertake their own research to further our understanding of the epidemiology of this important group of diseases.

REFERENCES

1. Ashford, N. A. 1976. *Crisis in the Workplace: Occupational Disease and Injury.* Cambridge, Mass.: MIT Press.
2. Cooper, B. S., and Rice, D. P. 1976. "The economic cost of illness revisited." *Social Security Bulletin* 39:21–36.
3. Haber, L. D. 1971. "Disability effects of chronic disease and impairments." *J. Chron. Dis.* 24:469–487.
4. Kelsey, J. L., Pastides, H., and Bisbee, G. E., Jr. 1978. *Musculo-skeletal Disorders: Their Frequency of Occurrence and Their Impact on the Population of the United States.* New York: Prodist.
5. Lenz, W. A. 1969. "Bone defects of the limbs—an overview." In *Birth Defects* (Original Article Series). D. Bergsona, ed. New York: March of Dimes, Vol. 5, p. 1.
6. Mebane, W. N. III. 1981. "Dog-walker's elbow." *New Engl. J. Med.* (Letter to the Editor) 304:613–614.
7. National Center for Health Statistics. 1973. *Limitation of Activity Due to Chronic Conditions, United States, 1969 and 1970.* Series 10, Number 80.
8. ———. 1974. *Chronic Conditions Causing Activity Limitation, United States, 1969–1970.* Series 10, Number 96.

9. ———. 1975. *Prevalence of Selected Impairments, United States, 1971.* Series 10, Number 99.

10. ———. 1976. *Hospital Discharges and Length of Stay: Short-Stay Hospitals, United States, 1972.* Series 10, Number 107.

11. ———. 1976. *Inpatient Utilization of Short-Stay Hospitals by Diagnosis, United States, 1973.* Series 13. Number 25.

12. ———. 1976. *Surgical Operations in Short-Stay Hospitals, United States, 1973.* Series 13, Number 24.

13. ———. 1976. *Vital Statistics of the United States, 1974. Volume II, Mortality, Part B* (HRA) 76-1115. Washington, U.S. Government Printing Office.

14. ———. 1977. *Limitation of Activity Due to Chronic Conditions, United States, 1974.* Series 10, Number 111.

15. ———. 1977. *State Estimates of Disability and Utilization of Medical Services, United States, 1969–1971.* DHEW Publication No. (HRA) 77-1241.

16. ———. 1979. *Acute Conditions. Incidence and Associated Disability, United States, July 1977–June 1978.* Series 10, Number 132.

17. ———. 1980. *The National Ambulatory Medical Care Survey 1977 Summary, United States, January–December, 1977.* Series 13, Number 44.

18. Shin, Y. 1977. "Variation in Hospital Costs and Product Heterogeneity." Thesis, Ph.D., Department of Epidemiology and Public Health, Yale University.

19. Thompson, M., Anderson, M., and Wood, P. H. N. 1974. "Locomotor disability— a study of need in an urban community." Abstract in *Brit. J. Prev. Soc. Med.* 28:70–71.

20. U.S. Social Security Administration. 1973. Social Security Disability Applicant Statistics. Unpublished Data.

21. ———. 1974. Office of Research and Statistics. *Medicare: Health Insurance for the Aged and Elderly, 1971. Discharges from Short-Stay Hospitals by Length of Stay for Selected Diagnoses, and Discharge Characteristics. Washington.*

22. White, K. "Life and death and medicine." 1973. *Sci. Am.* 229:23–33.

2 Congenital Malformations of the Musculoskeletal System

Congenital malformations of the musculoskeletal system are diagnosed among livebirths and stillbirths more frequently than defects of any other organ system (146). These malformations range from relatively mild anomalies such as extra fingers and toes to severe and disabling conditions such as spina bifida with involvement of the spinal canal.

Estimates of prevalence rates for all musculoskeletal conditions diagnosed at birth range from 3 to 10 percent depending on whether minor anomalies are counted as well as major abnormalities (16). Prevalence rates also vary considerably according to how the cases were identified and whether both stillbirths and livebirths or only livebirths are included. Table 2-1 shows prevalence rates per 1000 livebirths and stillbirths for the most common musculoskeletal anomalies as determined in the Collaborative Perinatal Project (92), the Center for Disease Control Congenital Malformation Surveillance Program for Metropolitan Atlanta (35), and the Center for Disease Control Congenital Malformation Surveillance Program for the United States (35). Although not based on a sample of births representative of any defined population, the data from the Collaborative Perinatal Project are derived from actual physical examinations performed on the infants at birth and at various intervals thereafter. The data from metropolitan Atlanta relate to a defined population, but are based on cases noted by physicians and hospitals. The statistics for the United States as a whole are based on large numbers of births, but depend upon hospital discharge abstracts from participating institutions. Thus, each source has its own particular strengths and weaknesses.

Table 2-1 Prevalence Rates per 1000 Livebirths and Stillbirths of the Most Frequently Occurring Musculoskeletal Anomalies, Three Sources of Data

Anomaly	Collaborative perinatal project 1959–1965[a] (92)				Metropolitan Atlanta July 1977–June 1978[b] (35)			United States July 1977–June 1978[c] (35)
	Total	White	Black	Puerto Rican	Total	White	Black	
Spina bifida								
With meningomyelocele	0.2*	0.2*	0.1*	0.6*	1.0	1.3	0.5	0.5*
Without central nervous system involvement	0.1*	0.2*	0.1*	—				
Clubfoot	3.8	3.6	4.2	2.6	3.8			2.3
Congenital dislocation of hip	1.8	3.2	0.5	2.0	0.9			3.5
Polydactyly	7.4	1.5	13.7	1.5	4.5	1.2	11.9	
Syndactyly	2.5	4.1	1.1	1.7	0.9			
Reduction deformities	1.6†	1.8†	1.5†	1.8†	0.8			0.4
Number of births	50,282	22,811	24,030	3,441	26,330			974,954

[a] A cohort of 50,282 mother-child pairs from 14 university-affiliated hospitals in the United States from 1959–1965 constitutes the study population. All children born after five lunar months of gestation are included. Infants were examined every day by pediatricians for the first week after delivery or weekly if the child stayed in the hospital longer. The mother was interviewed when the child was 4,8,12,18 and 24 months old, and then annually. If the child was taken to a physician or hospital, additional information was obtained from them. When a child reached one year of age, an extensive pediatric examination was given; 91 percent of the surviving children were examined at one year.

[b] Data include any liveborn or stillborn infant with a structural, chromosomal, or biochemical abnormality present at birth and diagnosed before the infant is one year of age and whose parents resided in Metropolitan Atlanta at the time of the birth. The registry is conducted in cooperation with hospitals and physicians of Metropolitan Atlanta.

[c] Data are obtained from discharge abstracts of all liveborn and stillborn infants in 1,130 hospitals participating in the Professional Activity Study (PAS).

*Includes only cases without anencephaly.

†Includes the categories (1) hypoplasia of limb or part and (2) absence of limb or part.

Throughout this chapter the variations in methods of case identification and criteria for inclusion limit the usefulness of comparisons from one study to another. In some studies, such criteria have not even been delineated. Despite these qualifications, useful epidemiologic information has been obtained on the epidemiology of these common congenital musculoskeletal conditions.

SPINA BIFIDA

Spina bifida is a defect of closure of the bony spinal canal. It has long been believed that this results from failure of the posterior parts of the vertebral segment to fuse during early fetal development, specifically in the third to fourth week of fetal life (158). Recently it has been suggested (83) that neural tube defects such as spina bifida may occur because of overdistension and rupture of the tube after normal closure. If this hypothesis were to receive further support, etiologic studies would take new directions (152).

Spina bifida occurs in two forms: spina bifida occulta and spina bifida cystica. Spina bifida occulta has no associated abnormality of the spinal cord or meninges, seldom exhibits symptoms, and the diagnosis generally is not made unless X-rays taken for other reasons reveal a defect in the bony spinal canal. Spina bifida occulta will not be considered further here, except to note that its frequency of occurrence in X-rays taken for other reasons has been reported to range from 5 to 36 percent (71). In spina bifida cystica, the contents of the spinal canal are exposed on the body surface, the meninges may herniate and produce a fluid-filled sac (a meningocele), the meninges and spinal nerve roots may be exposed (a meningomyelocele), or nerve tissue in the primitive state may appear as an open plaque on the back (a myelocele). Spina bifida cystica frequently occurs in association with anencephaly, which is a defect of closure at the anterior end of the spinal canal such that all or part of the cranial vault and cerebral hemispheres are missing. These two neural defects together are responsible for more stillbirths and early infant deaths than any other malformation (201).

Most infants with anencephaly are stillborn, and those who are born alive survive only briefly. From 30 to 50 percent of infants with spina bifida cystica without anencephaly are also stillborn (62). Among those born alive, only about 60 percent survive for one year, despite improvements in surgical techniques (176). Almost all who do survive have some

degree of handicap resulting from such physical impairments as para-
lyzed legs, hip deformities, knee deformities, foot deformities, spinal curvature, and incontinence, and sometimes mental impairment as well.
Many undergo multiple operations for these problems.

Numerous studies have been undertaken of the epidemiology of spina
bifida and anencephaly, but only a summary of the current state of
knowledge will be presented. The reader is referred to a more detailed
review by J. M. Elwood and J. H. Elwood (65) for further information.
Most epidemiologic studies of spina bifida have been done in conjunction
with anencephaly since the two conditions tend to occur in the same individuals more frequently than would be expected by chance (130,172),
many of their epidemiologic characteristics are similar (95,136,141), they
cluster in the same families (31), and their embryonic origin is presumed
to be similar (158). Therefore, except where noted, most of the findings
presented here apply to both conditions.

Frequency

Estimates of the prevalence rate of spina bifida at birth vary because of
true geographic variation in underlying incidence rates during early pregnancy and because of different diagnostic criteria and possible variations
in miscarriage and abortion rates of affected fetuses (62,75,178). The
Birth Defects Monitoring Program (BDMP) of the Centers for Disease
Control (34), which includes both stillbirths and livebirths, reported a
prevalence rate of 5.0 per 10,000 births in the United States in 1979 for
spina bifida diagnosed at birth without anencephaly; rates reported from
other sources in the United States were shown in Table 1-1. The prevalence rate for anencephaly diagnosed at birth with or without spina
bifida was 3.6 per 10,000 in 1979 as reported by the BDMP (33). Rates
of neural tube defects are considerably higher among embryos and fetuses
aborted early in pregnancy (45,128,162,179). Creasy and Alberman (45)
suggest that about half of the fetuses affected with anencephaly and spina
bifida spontaneously abort by 27 weeks, compared to 14 percent of unaffected fetuses. Even higher proportions were reported in the Japanese
data of Nishimura (162).

Geographic Variation

Prevalence rates for spina bifida at birth vary considerably among countries (see Figure 2-1), and most investigators feel that much of the vari-

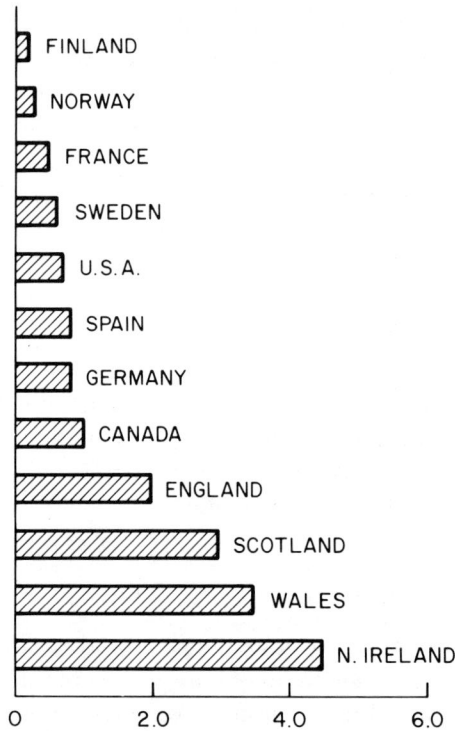

Figure 2-1 Prevalence of spina bifida per 1000 total births.

Source: Scrimgeour and Cockburn (189).

ation reflects true differences in prevalence at birth. In a World Health Organization sponsored study of 24 large maternity hospitals in 16 countries (201), the highest prevalence rates for spina bifida were found in Belfast, Northern Ireland (4.3 per 1000 births). Most countries had rates of 0.3 to 1.5 per 1000. Areas with low rates (1.0 per 1000 or less) include Israel, Scandinavia, Africa, Asia, and South America (87,111,189, 194,201). In the United States and also in Canada, mortality from spina bifida has appeared in the past to be highest in the East and lowest in the West (61,65,93), but more recent data from the Centers for Disease Control (33) do not show this geographical gradient in the United States. Within the United Kingdom, the highest rates are found in the north and west, with the peak rates found in Northern Ireland and Wales (28,57,59,203). Within countries higher rates are generally found in urban than in rural areas (4,95).

Trends with Time

Long-term trends in prevalence and mortality rates for neural tube defects have been noted, but they differ from place to place, and no causative agents have been identified. In Boston, Massachusetts, Providence, Rhode Island (142,155), and Rochester, New York (17), reported rates of anencephaly and spina bifida increased from 1915 to 1932, and then declined. Consistent with these trends, in upstate New York a decline in prevalence was noted from 1945 through at least 1971 (85,104, 106), and the BDMP has noted a slight decrease in prevalence of spina bifida in the United States from 7.2 per 10,000 births in 1970 to 5.0 per 10,000 births in 1979 (34). In Canada, annual mortality rates for anencephaly and spina bifida peaked around 1950, and have generally decreased since then, with a small increase around 1960–62. However, there are exceptions to this overall trend in that no long-term decline in mortality was observed in British Columbia (61,62). Also, a decline in mortality rates since 1943–44 in Ontario paralleled the trend observed in the northeastern United States, whereas in Quebec, mortality rates peaked around 1951–54 and then decreased (65). Elwood and Elwood (65) think that this decline started too early to be attributable to improved methods of surgery introduced in the late 1950s, so that the trends in mortality rates probably reflect trends in prevalence rates at birth.

   In contrast, in England and Wales (183) mortality rates for spina bifida and anencephaly increased for nearly a century until 1942–43, then decreased until 1948–49, increased until 1954–55, and subsequently decreased again. Prevalence rates for neural tube defects in Birmingham, England, have paralleled these trends from the 1940s to the 1960s (129). Since 1960, mortality rates from anencephaly have been relatively constant in England and Wales (65), but local variations are again apparent. In Dublin, Ireland, the rates peaked during 1960–61, but this temporary increase was not observed in the country as a whole (58). Trends in neural tube stillbirths and neonatal deaths similar to those in England and Wales have been observed from 1950 to 1974 in New South Wales, Australia (76), and a decrease in prevalence rates of neural tube defects in Israel has been noted from 1958 to 1964 (156).

   Seasonal trends in prevalence and mortality have also been apparent, although variation from place to place is again found. A winter excess of births of spina bifida (25,130,131) and anencephaly cases (54,55,57,147) has been noted by some, but not all, investigators in England, Wales, and Northern Ireland, suggesting the existence of an as yet unidentified teratogenic agent acting in spring and early summer. In North America seasonal trends have in general not been noted (65). In New South Wales, Australia, one study (76) detected an excess of anencephalic and spina bifida births in spring, while a study in Victoria, Australia (44), showed no particular seasonal variation. In Israel, too, no significant seasonal variation has been noted (156). Above and beyond the secular and seasonal trends, "epidemics" of spina bifida and anencephaly from time to time in certain localities in certain years have occurred (5,107,190). However, no explanations for the "epidemics" have been found.

Demographic Characteristics

One of the few known differences between the epidemiology of spina bifida and that of anencephaly is the sex ratio. In Western countries, females are affected more frequently with both conditions than are males, but the ratio of females to males is less for spina bifida (1.3 to 1) than for anencephaly (2 to 1) (28,131). The female-to-male ratio is highest for anencephaly where its prevalence is greatest (156,203), and the ratio is much higher during epidemic than nonepidemic periods (184). However, in Japan, Taiwan, and Singapore, the proportion of males among those affected with anencephaly is close to 50 percent even in areas where the prevalence of anencephaly is relatively high, while for spina bifida, the percentage of males is similar to the approximately 40 percent found in Western countries (65). Secular variations in anencephaly mortality rates have also been noted in some places to be more marked for females than males (106,130,184), although in Canada, this has not been seen (65). These observations have led to the suggestion that certain unknown environmental risk factors for anencephaly affect female embryos to a greater extent than male embryos (184). For spina bifida, however, the sex ratio has remained relatively constant over both time and place (65).

Considerable differences in the frequency of neural tube defects have been observed from one racial or ethnic group to another. Leck (130) reported that the highest rates of neural tube defects are found in Caucasians, with lower rates in Mongoloids and Negroes. Rates for blacks appear to be low regardless of location (190). In Australia part-aboriginal children have been found to be at higher risk than white Australians (76). In North America low rates occur among Jews and high rates among Irish (95,141,157). Conflicting results have been reported regarding the extent to which rates in migrants approach those of the country of immigration (131,190). Elwood and Elwood (65) find that in Canada both place of residence at the time of birth and maternal ethnic origin have independent effects on the anencephaly mortality rate. Considering all the evidence together they conclude that prevalence rates of neural tube defects in Caucasian populations are influenced by the environment to which the migrants have moved, and that rates in the second or third generations approach those of the new country. However, in black and Oriental populations prevalence rates apparently change only slightly after migration. Why there should be different effects among migrants of different races is not known.

Many studies in a variety of localities have documented that the highest risks for spina bifida and anencephaly occur in lower social classes (9,54,59,74,76,95,157,195). Whether certain parental occupations are associated with elevated risks has not been determined (65).

Birth Order and Maternal Age

Knowledge of effects of birth order and maternal age is still evolving. Most cross-sectional studies have shown high rates to be associated with first births, low rates with second births, and increasing rates with births after the second, such that rates with five or more previous births are as high as rates among first born (28,54,62,65,76,95,98,157,170,172). Similarly, rates found in cross-sectional studies are high among women under 20 years of age and over 35 years of age, with lower rates at intermediate ages, especially in the 20 to 24 years of age group (28,31,95,98,170,185). In some studies the birth order effect has appeared to be stronger than the maternal age effect (98,172), while in others the effects of maternal age and birth order appear to be independent (72,74,95,170).

Cross-sectional studies, however, can be misleading, and it has been recognized that maternal age and birth order associations may be due to a cohort effect (98). Recent reports have in fact indicated that within a maternal birth cohort, the prevalence of anencephaly and spina bifida actually decreases slightly with increasing maternal age (62,102–104). The existence of a cohort effect suggested to one author (103) that factors operating early in the life of the mother may be more important than those to which she is exposed during pregnancy. On the other hand, J. M. Elwood et al. (67) found that if place, year and season of birth, and maternal ethnic origin of anencephaly cases were all taken into account, there was no overall association of risk with maternal age. They did find a decrease in risk for anencephaly with increasing number of previous livebirths and an increase in risk with greater number of previous stillbirths and infant deaths. A case-control study by J. M. Elwood and McBride (66) confirmed that within sibships, the risk for neural tube defects decreases with increasing birth rank, and also that affected infants tend to come from families with larger than expected numbers of children. An especially high risk was associated with the first birth, and it has been suggested (65) that the effect of other risk factors may vary according to whether a woman is giving birth to her first child or a later child. For instance, it was found that although there is no overall association between maternal age and anencephaly when other factors were taken into account, among first births the average risk decreased with increasing maternal age while in later births, the risk increased. Thus, the birth order and maternal age effects are more complicated than previously realized, and further research is needed.

Suggested Etiologic Agents

Neural tube defect mortality and prevalence rates have thus been found to be correlated with several variables. Consideration of these patterns has led to the formulation of hypotheses about etiologic roles for such factors as softness of water supply, exposure to metals, diet, maternal hyperthermia, heredity, fetus-fetus interaction, and effects of previous pregnancies. Although at present there is no definitive evidence for a causal role for any of these factors, the evidence that does exist will briefly be reviewed.

In general, higher rates of anencephaly and spina bifida have been found in areas that have softer water supplies than in areas that have harder water supplies in the United Kingdom (72,137) and the United States (72), but not in New South Wales, Australia (76). In Canada (63), rates are just slightly lower in localities with hard water supplies. The associations with water softness have led to interest in the possible effects of certain metals that tend to be present in soft water. For instance, soft acid waters would be likely to dissolve more lead from the pipes through which the water passes (72), suggesting that lead might be an etiologic agent. J. M. Elwood (63) noted an association between low magnesium concentrations and mortality rates from neural tube defects in Canada, but did not attach any causal significance to this correlation. Insufficient iodine in drinking water has also been suggested as a cause (18), but it was not found to be related to increased prevalence of neural tube defects in a study in Rochester, New York (18).

Although the possibility of an etiologic role for water remains an area of interest, local fluctuations and differences in water hardness by place and time do not appear to be related to the prevalence of anencephaly and spina bifida (18,78). Results of a recent case-control study provide little support for an etiologic role for trace elements in tap water (188). It is generally felt that the geographic correlations with water softness are most likely attributable to some as yet undetermined secondary factor (137).

Experiments in animals have shown that a variety of dietary factors can influence the occurrence of neural tube defects (65), and a possible role for dietary factors has also received attention in humans. For instance, an unbalanced diet (176) could explain the social class gradient. Renwick (174,175) suggested that some factor associated with blighted potatoes increased the risk for anencephaly and spina bifida. He based this view largely on changes in prevalence rates over time in certain geographic areas that appeared to him to be related to severity of potato blight. However, this has not been confirmed by other investigators, and case-control studies provide no support for the hypothesis (42,58,59, 68,143,180,197,200). Sever and Emanuel (191) have hypothesized, on the basis of animal experiments and on the basis of some characteristics of the descriptive epidemiology of neural tube defects, that maternal zinc deficiency should be considered as a possible etiologic factor, but no epidemiologic studies to evaluate this hypothesis have yet been undertaken.

Knox (121,122) has correlated data on diet in England and Wales with stillbirth and infant death rates from neural tube defects over time, taking into account both seasonal and secular trends. In light of the temporal correlations, geographic patterns, and evidence from animal experiments, he felt that cured meats, which result in exposure to nitrosamines and other nitrosocompounds, should receive further study. Unfortunately, no further study has been undertaken, and this hypothesis remains untested.

Fedrick (73) noted that the social class differences in prevalence of neural tube defects, the worldwide geographic variation, and to a certain extent the temporal variation were correlated with amount of tea drinking. In a case-control study she found that the risk of neural tube defects was in fact increased in women who drank three or more cups of tea per day, but there was no gradient in risk below or above this amount; also, the elevated risk was seen only in women who resided in areas of high or medium prevalence, suggesting that perhaps an effect of tea occurred mainly in localities with soft water. It would thus seem that further studies of maternal tea drinking are warranted.

More recently, Smithells et al. (199) have reported that women who had previously given birth to infants with neural tube defects had lower subsequent rates for these defects if they were given multivitamin supplements. Because this was not a randomized trial, however, self-selection remains a possibility, and this is yet another area that needs more study.

Episodes of maternal hyperthermia have been considered as etiologic factors. Miller et al. (150) reported from a small case-control study that mothers of anencephalic infants were more likely to have had a febrile illness or a history of sauna bathing during the presumed time of anterior neural groove closure than mothers of control infants. They cited confirmatory results from animal studies (198) and also subsequently received support from another case-control study (88). Although these case-control studies were not rigorously conducted and had the possible problem of memory bias (133), and although Finland with its high use of sauna baths has very low rates of neural tube defects (87), this hypothesis should be more carefully tested.

Familial aggregation of cases of spina bifida and anencephaly has generated considerable interest. It has long been recognized that 3 to 5 percent of siblings of affected infants also have spina bifida or anencephaly, a risk that is about ten times higher than infants in the general population (29,31,127,135,141,156). Elwood and Elwood (65) have pointed out that the sibling risk is greater in the United Kingdom than in the United States or the rest of Europe, the average risks being 4.6 percent, 2.8 percent, and 2.8 percent, respectively. It appears that risks to offspring of parents with spina bifida are of a similar magnitude to the risks in siblings of an affected child, and that this risk is similar for affected fathers and affected mothers (30). The extent to which this familial aggregation is attributable to heredity or to exposure to common environmental agents is an issue that has generated some controversy. Although firm evidence is lacking, most investigators feel that to the extent that heredity is involved, the mode of inheritance is likely to be polygenic (29,31,107,127), and that the environmental component is probably more important than the genetic one (65,130,201). A form of cytoplasmic inheritance proposed by Nance (159) has not been studied further.

Whether recurrence rates are higher in full sibs than in half sibs and in full sibs than in dizygotic twins is not at the present time clear (31,107,145,230). However, Knox (120) called attention to the apparent infrequency with which either member of a monozygous twin pair is affected, to the rarity of concordance for neural tube defects in dizygous twins, and to the excess of like-sexed pairs among the dizygous twin pairs in which one member is affected.

On the basis of the familial aggregation, the twin data, and the sex ratio, Knox (120) proposed that the occurrence of neural tube defects may be explained in part by a fetus-fetus interaction based on a sex-linked mode of inheritance. In the interaction, one fetus is destroyed and the other is left with a neural tube defect. Neural tube defects in discordant twins could be explained by an interaction involving initial triplets. Knox (123) found that this hypothesis at least roughly explained many of the disparate features of the epidemiology of neural tube defects, and further proposed that about one-third of cases might be explained by an interaction between residual trophoblastic material from a previous normal pregnancy in which the infant was of the opposite sex from the fetus who developed a neural tube defect.

Promising though Knox's hypothesis was, it was consistent with some but not all of the epidemiologic observations. Clarke et al. (41), for instance, found no evidence of an altered sex ratio among sibs born immediately before an affected child, but they as well as Field and Kerr (77) did find more miscarriages and stillbirths in the pregnancy before the birth of the child with a neural tube defect than in the births after the affected child. Since retention of pathologic trophoblastic material would be more likely to occur after a miscarriage than after a normal delivery, they conclude that this finding is consistent with the hypothesis that retention of trophoblastic material is a risk factor for anencephaly and spina bifida. Gardiner et al. (82) and Laurence and Roberts (128) confirmed these results, but the latter authors as well as James (101) feel that the lack of correlation of the length of the interval between miscarriage and conception with pregnancy outcome suggests other explanations. One such explanation would be that miscarriages are a manifestation rather than a cause of neural tube defects, since many miscarried or aborted fetuses may themselves be affected. Thus, although the fetus-fetus interaction is in many ways an attractive hypothesis, it is by no means widely accepted.

Numerous other possible risk factors have been proposed. Infectious agents such as the influenza virus have been suggested, but a careful review of available evidence (140) provides little support for a role for the influenza virus. Other infectious agents have not been well studied, and there is little evidence of time-space clustering (193,210). It is possible that if infectious diseases are associated with an increased risk, the relevant infection occurred much earlier in a woman's life than during her pregnancy (65,103). No convincing evidence of a possible association of drug use and exposure to anaesthetic agents during pregnancy with anencephaly and spina bifida has so far been found (65). Also, several studies have shown little or no increase in risk of neural tube malformation among women who have been exposed to oral contraceptives in the period immediately before or after conception or to hormonal pregnancy tests (23,90,149,164,186). Any effect of cigarette smoking is likely to be small (65), and midcycle abstinence from sexual intercourse was not found to be an important factor (125).

Archer (6) correlated mortality rates from anencephaly with horizontal geomagnetic flux, proposing that where there is lower geomagnetic flux (nearer to magnetic north), there is higher exposure to cosmic radiation, and that this in turn increases the risk for anencephaly. However, this hypothesis has been found to be inconsistent with most available data (64). A deficiency of human chorionic gonadotropin (HCG) has been suggested as an explanation for the sex ratio and the rates in twins (105,106), but this has been neither confirmed nor refuted.

Summary

Although much is known about the distribution of anencephaly and spina bifida in the population, and although there are in all likelihood many contributory causes, not a single generally accepted causal mechanism has been identified. Most epidemiologic work to date can be classified as hypothesis generating, and rigorous testing of these hypotheses is needed. The most promising hypotheses that could be tested by means of case-control studies concern the possible etiologic roles of maternal tea drinking, exposure to nitrosocompounds, exposure to lead, hyperthermia around the third to fourth week of pregnancy, and adverse outcomes of previous pregnancies. In the course of these studies, information could be sought about possible risk factors to which a mother might have been exposed earlier in her life. The possibility that different risk factors are important in different geographic areas also needs to be kept in mind.

CONGENITAL DISLOCATION OF THE HIP

In congenital dislocation of the hip, there is complete or partial displacement of the femoral head upward out of the acetabulum; partial displacement is sometimes referred to as congenital subluxation of the hip. In about 80 percent of cases the diagnosis is made upon examination shortly after birth. In the other 20 percent the diagnosis is made later, particularly when the child starts to walk. It is known that in some of the "late-diagnosis" cases there were no clinical signs of hip disorders on examination immediately after birth. Although it is possible that the screening tests used at birth are not as sensitive as desired, it seems likely that some cases do in fact develop after birth, since some late-diagnosis cases had been given very thorough examinations at birth (21).

About half of the hips found to be unstable at birth become stable spontaneously within three weeks (112). The effectiveness of treatment of more severe forms depends to a large extent on early diagnosis and treatment. If proper treatment is not given, the affected leg may be shorter, the child may limp, surgical intervention may be needed, and osteoarthrosis of the hip is likely to occur in adulthood. There is some evidence that even slight congenital abnormalities in the development of the hip joint can lead to later osteoarthrosis (112,205,214).

The frequency of congenital dislocation of the hip varies considerably from one geographic area to another. Rates between 1 and 10 per 1000 births have been found in most North American and Western European populations and in Israel, Australia, and New Zealand (10,21,34,43,52, 91,148,167,171,212). Much greater rates ranging from 10 per 1000 to as high as around 100 per 1000 have been reported among the Navajo, Apache, and Cree-Ojibwa Indians of North America (124,168,213), the Lapps (84), and in Hungary (48), northern Italy (204), Brittany (229) and the Faroe Islands (161). Congenital dislocation of the hip is rare, on the other hand, among blacks in South Africa, the West Indies, and Uganda (53,86,211), as well as among Chinese living in Hong Kong (94).

It has been reported that in some areas, including the United States (34), the occurrence of congenital dislocation of the hip has been rising in recent years. In most areas this has been attributed to more extensive screening after birth, more awareness on the part of physicians, and better reporting to registries (15,19,21,132). The greater intensity of screening and greater awareness by physicians may in fact in some instances lead to diagnosis and perhaps treatment of hip problems that would have stabilized by themselves if left untreated (132). However, in Israel an increase in frequency has been noted over the years 1966 to 1975 despite the use of consistent screening policies and diagnostic criteria during this period (118,119). The reasons for this increase are not known.

In most areas, females are affected more frequently than males by about a 6 to 1 ratio (21,36,37,52,148,171,181,219,226). Also, rates are higher in whites than blacks (26,53,86,181, 211).

The percentage of cases that are affected bilaterally varies in different

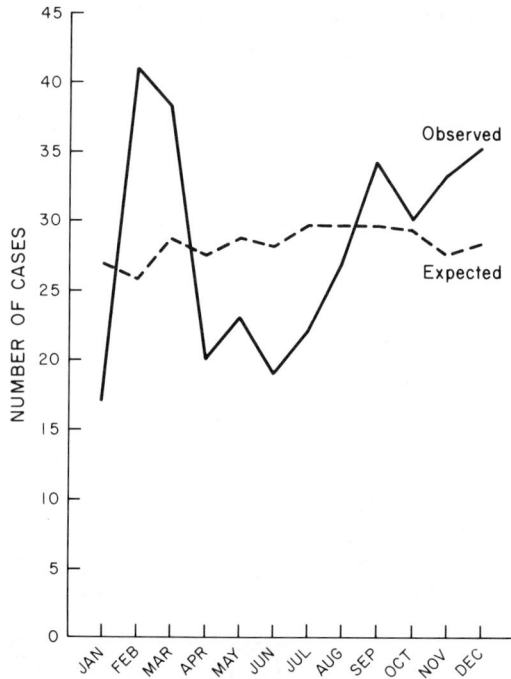

Figure 2-2   Distribution of observed and expected cases of congenital dislocation of the hip by month of birth.

Source: Robinson (181).

studies, but among unilateral cases, the left hip is affected two to three
times more frequently than the right in both sexes (20,21,47,
153,167,171,181,196). Most studies of seasonal variation suggest a
greater than expected number of cases among those born in late fall and
winter than in summer (see Figure 2-2) (36,37,47,171,181,219,226),
although this has not been noted in all areas (10,167,168,229).

It is well established that infants with congenital dislocation of the hip
are more likely to have been born by breech delivery than other infants
(3,21,27,47,52,79,148,153,167,171,181,196,226), and some investigators
have found that breech delivery is a more important risk factor in males
than in females (see Table 2-2) (3,4,148,171,181). The higher percentage
of congenital dislocation of the hip among firstborn infants is attributable
to their having a higher frequency of breech deliveries (21,47). It has also
been reported that, on the average, infants with congenital dislocation of
the hip have had longer gestation periods than other infants (47).

Table 2-2 Percentage of Deliveries Which Are Breech among Infants with
Congenital Dislocation of the Hip by Birth Rank and Sex

Birth rank	Sex	Number of deliveries	Percentage of deliveries which are breech
1	Male	10	30.0
	Female	65	21.5
2 or greater	Male	13	53.8
	Female	73	4.1
Total	Male	23	43.5
	Female	138	12.3

Source: Record and Edwards (171).

Familial aggregation of cases has been repeatedly found
(21,171,181,219,226). Studies in twins suggest that both heredity and
environment contribute to the familial aggregation (32). It is worth not-
ing that in dogs, in whom congenital dislocation of the hip has been
extensively studied, it also has been concluded that both environment and
heredity are involved, probably through multifactorial inheritance (171).
In humans, there is some evidence that abnormalities in the development
of the acetabulum from polygenic inheritance and laxity of the joint capsule from monogenic inheritance are etiologic factors (32,49,225,226).
Two forms of familial joint laxity have been hypothesized, one a persistent form affecting boys more than girls (27,32,49) and the other a transient form resulting from temporary elevation of hormone levels in newborn girls (32,215). Although shallow acetabula and laxity may indeed
be predisposing factors, modes of inheritance are not yet established.
Opinions also differ as to whether acetabular dysplasia predisposes to
congenital dislocation of the hip or whether dislocation is the cause of
acetabular dysplasia, with most evidence supporting the latter view (21).
Furthermore, it has been suggested that lack of support from the ligament
of the head of the femur rather than from the joint capsule contributes to
susceptibility to congenital dislocation of the hip (46).

Levels of estrogens have been studied in newborns with dislocated hips,
since it has been hypothesized that the seasonal distribution of congenital
dislocation of the hip and the excess of cases with long periods of gestation
could be attributed to hormonal factors that contribute both to long ges-

tation and to laxity of the hip joint (4,47). However, studies of whether estrogen levels are in fact higher than expected in newborns with congenital dislocation of the hip have yielded contradictory results (1,4,169,209), possibly because of different methods of hormone assay. Studies using the more refined methods currently available might resolve some of these differences.

Position in utero probably plays an etiologic role. It is likely, for instance, that breech position in utero elongates the hip joint capsule of the ligament by persistent upward pressure of the greater trochanter (110). Also, breech position in utero may have been produced by a factor interfering with leg folding, which would make version difficult and which might predispose to congenital dislocation of the hip as well (217). In addition, the intrauterine position may be at least partly responsible for the side on which the dislocation occurs. It has been reported (51), although apparently not confirmed, that the fetus lies with its back toward its mother's left side about twice as often as toward her right side, and that the posterior leg is more likely to be dislocated than the anterior one, regardless of whether presentation is breech or vertex. This observation would be consistent with the greater frequency of the disorder in the left hip than the right.

In one study of "unselected newborns" (26), the acetabular angle (which is an indicator of the extent of upward tilting of the acetabular roof) was found on the average to be slightly greater in the left hip than in the right hip at birth, six months, and one year. Although the average differences were perhaps too small to be of clinical significance, a greater acetabular angle in the left hip could contribute to the predominance of dislocations in the left hip. Also, there is one report that amniocentesis is associated with an increased risk for congenital dislocation of the hip (222).

Postnatal factors to which infants are exposed have also been considered in the etiology of this disorder. In particular, possible stresses on the hip from clothing or from methods of carrying infants in certain cultures have been postulated to be etiologically involved, since these might explain the seasonal distribution in frequency (171) and the high rates in some geographic areas (48,84,168,211). However, studies in some of the areas of particularly high or low frequency have not confirmed this postulate (168,211), and it is unlikely that such practices are of etiologic significance. It has also been hypothesized, but not studied epidemiologically, that the practice that some physicians have of holding the infant by the heel in an inverted position to allow drainage of mucus could lead to dislocation in infants who already have lax hips (46).

Recently, studies have suggested etiologic differences in those congenital dislocations diagnosed just after birth and those diagnosed later. Although familial aggregation of cases occurs in both types, breech delivery and long gestation appear to be stronger risk factors for early-diagnosed cases, while the excess of cases in late fall is more marked for late-diagnosed cases. Late-diagnosed cases tend to have shorter gestation periods and lower birth weights (21,47).

In summary, congenital dislocation of the hip occurs more frequently in females than males, affects whites more often than blacks, is found in the left hip more often than the right, occurs with high frequency in breech deliveries, in infants with long gestation periods, and in families in which one member has already been affected, and shows considerable variation in frequency from one geographic area to another. However, much remains to be learned about possible modes of inheritance and about the specific factors that produce the variation in frequency from one subgroup of the population to another. Position in utero and ligamentous or capsular laxity are probably predisposing factors that explain some of the descriptive epidemiology, but other characteristics, such as the geographic and seasonal variations in frequency, remain to be explained. Also, hormonal involvement remains an attractive etiologic hypothesis since elevated estrogen levels could bring about laxity in the structures supporting the head of the femur and since animal experiments support an etiologic role for hormones. Finally, confirmation is needed of the recent reports that risk factors for cases diagnosed at birth may be to some degree different from those diagnosed later.

CLUBFOOT

The term clubfoot is used to describe several congenital malformations of the foot that are considered clinically and possibly etiologically distinct. The three most commonly described forms are talipes equinovarus, metatarsus varus, and talipes calcaneovalgus. Talipes equinovarus, also called "common clubfoot" and "congenital idiopathic clubfoot," is shown in Figure 2-3. In this type, the forefoot is turned inward, the heel is tucked upward, the plantar surface faces medially, and there is flexion of the plantar surface of the forefoot and ankle. This condition is almost always diagnosed at birth, and despite the abnormal position and the impaired function, all normal structures are present without pathological changes. In metatarsus varus, the inner border of the foot is off the ground with the sole turned inward. This is more readily corrected than talipes equi-

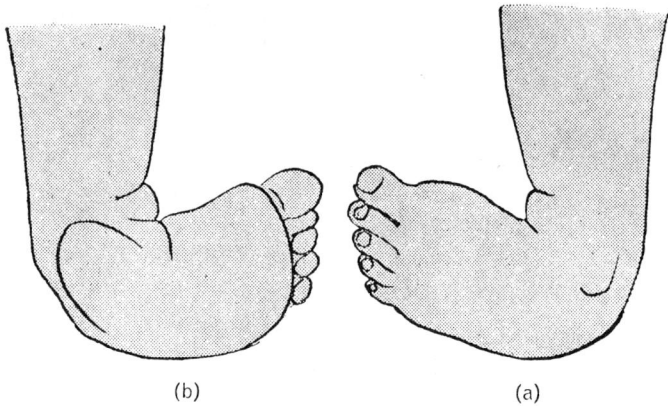

(b)   (a)

Figure 2-3 Appearance of congenital talipes equinovarus. (*a*) Anterior view. (*b*) Posterior view.

Source: Aston (7).

novarus. It is frequently not noted at birth, and may remain undetected until one to three months after birth or occasionally not until the child starts to walk. In talipes calcaneovalgus, the heel is turned outward from the midline of the body and the front part of the foot is elevated. This anomaly is considered very mild and is often self-correcting. While some epidemiologic studies have included other foot malformations in the category of clubfoot, these three types, and in particular talipes equinovarus, have received the most attention. In fact, because the other two clinical types are frequently self-correcting or easily corrected, many studies have focused just on the more severe form, talipes equinovarus.

Estimated prevalence rates at birth for all types of clubfoot deformities have ranged from 0.8 per 1000 livebirths to 4.4 per 1000 livebirths (38,96,173,224). In a study that also included stillbirths, Alberman (2) reported a prevalence rate of 14.1 per 1000 births for any type of foot deformity. Comparisons of rates from one geographic area to another or from one study to another have been of limited value thus far because of differences in case definition and in thoroughness of case ascertainment. Also, some studies include only livebirths while others include stillbirths or fetal deaths.

About 55 percent of cases of talipes equinovarus are bilateral. Among unilateral cases, the right foot is affected slightly more often than the left in the ratio of about 1.2 to 1 (40,117,165). Metatarsus varus occurs bilaterally somewhat more often than does talipes equinovarus, with talipes calcaneovalgus occupying an intermediate position.

Clubfoot has been reported to occur together with other congenital abnormalities in the same infants more frequently than expected by chance, although the proportion of cases in which this is seen and the types of abnormalities with which the different types of clubfoot are associated vary from one study to another (2,117,223,224,228). One type of abnormality that Wynne-Davies (223) found in many cases of clubfoot was a generalized joint laxity that she hypothesized might make an infant more susceptible to uterine pressure at some critical stage of intrauterine development.

Talipes equinovarus has consistently been observed about twice as frequently in males as in females (12,22,117,165,166,223,228), whereas females have higher frequencies of metatarsus varus and talipes calcaneovalgus (2,223,224). Wynne-Davies (223), for instance, reported a male-to-female ratio of 0.8 to 1 for metatarus varus and 0.6 to 1 for talipes calcaneovalgus. One study suggests that the male to female ratio for talipes equinovarus is higher among cases without a family history of clubfoot (165).

Within the United States, whites are at greater risk for clubfoot in general than nonwhites (39,192). Polynesian populations, including native Hawaiians (38,202) and Maoris in New Zealand (12,56,96), have high prevalence rates. Whether risks for clubfoot vary according to social class has apparently not been evaluated.

The epidemiologic characteristic of clubfoot that has received the most attention is the familial aggregation of cases. Most investigators have reported higher prevalence rates of clubfoot among relatives of index cases than among the general population and have found that the rates vary by the degree-of-relationship (22,117,165,173,223,228). Palmer (165), for instance, noted that compared to the general population there was a 21-fold increased risk for talipes equinovarus among first-degree relatives of cases with talipes equinovarus, a five-fold increase among second degree relatives, and a two-fold increase in third degree relatives. There is one report (228) that first-degree relatives of female cases are at particularly high risk. Idelberger (97) found that of the 174 twin pairs included in his study, the concordance rate among monozygotic twins was 33 percent, in contrast to 3 percent among the dizygotic twins. Palmer (165) estimated that if one child in a family was affected with talipes equinovarus, the probability of a subsequent child being born with talipes equinovarus was about 3 percent, while Reimann (173) reported that 1 to 2 percent of siblings of cases had clubfoot if neither parent had been affected, as compared to 3 percent if one or both parents had been affected. Although most studies have focused on talipes equinovarus, relatives of cases with the other forms of clubfoot are also at increased risk for these deformities (223). A higher prevalence of a variety of other congenital malformations, including hydrocephalus, spina bifida, anencephaly and congenital heart disease, was noted by Alberman (2) among older sibs of talipes equinovarus cases, but this result has not been evaluated by other investigators.

Findings on possible associations between the occurrence of clubfoot and young maternal age or low birth order have been somewhat contradictory (2,12,40,165,173,223,224). A few investigators have reported increased risks for one or more forms of clubfoot among infants with young mothers or among firstborn infants (2,39,165,223,224), although most have not tried to separate effects of young maternal age from effects of low parity. Since an increased frequency among firstborn might be expected because of the tighter uterine musculature in primiparous women (2,223), it would seem that primiparity as a risk factor merits further study. While this hypothesis suggests that there should be an excess of twins among cases of clubfoot, no such excess has been found (40).

Other maternal factors reported in single studies as being related to one or other type of clubfoot but that have not been evaluated in other studies are amniocentesis (222), thyroid disorders (144), smallpox vaccinations during the first trimester (154), use of salicylate preparations during the first trimester (176), and amobarbital exposure prenatally (92). Other thermal, chemical, nutritive, hormonal, and infectious agents have also been suggested (173), but as yet no studies have adequately tested these hypotheses in humans. Recently, based on observations in embryos, fetuses, and stillborn infants, a vascular abnormality causing localized ischemia has been suggested in the etiology of clubfoot (8), but this too needs further evaluation.

It is generally accepted that both environmental and genetic factors are involved in the etiology of clubfoot. Also, it is agreed that the skeletal and neuromuscular changes in foot structure that accompany clubfoot are consequences rather than causes of clubfoot (14,99,173,216). However, little agreement exists about genetic mechanisms or environmental causes. Various genetic mechanisms have been proposed, including autosomal recessive, sex-linked recessive, autosomal dominant with incomplete penetrance, and multifactorial inheritance; it is generally felt that the most likely mode of inheritance is multifactorial (40,165). Among environmental factors, the one that has received perhaps the most interest is intrauterine pressure at a critical stage of fetal development (2,165), and it would be useful to have more information on this hypothesis from animal models. As further epidemiologic studies are undertaken on other suggested risk factors, attention should be paid to the possibly differing etiologies of the individual forms of clubfoot.

OTHER MALFORMATIONS OF THE EXTREMITIES

Syndactyly

In syndactyly, two or more fingers or toes are partially or completely grown together (see Figure 2-4). The condition may be corrected by surgically separating the fingers and using skin grafts for repair. Several classification systems for syndactyly have been proposed, most of which consider the following characteristics: (1) whether the attachment consists of a webbing only of skin between digits (the simplest form) or involves the underlying soft tissues and abnormal fusion of the phalangeal bones as well (50,69,80,114,187), (2) whether or not the extent of the attach-

Figure 2-4   Syndactyly.

Source: MacAusland and Mayo (138).

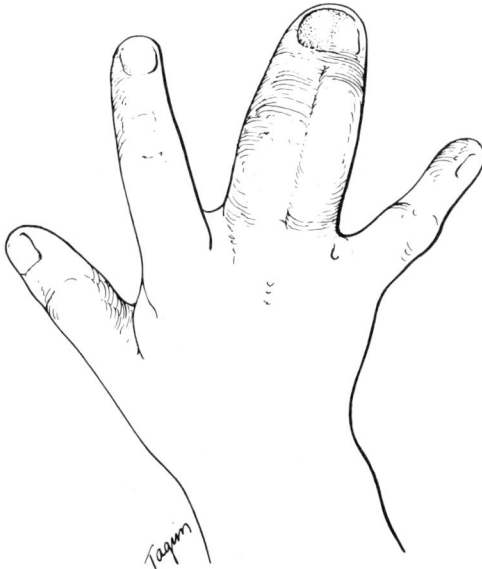

ment extends to the ends of the digits (80,114), and (3) whether the attachment is present as an isolated anomaly or as part of a syndrome (187). Even if not part of a specific syndrome, syndactyly frequently occurs in conjunction with a variety of other congenital malformations (11,13,50,69,80,92,115,116,139,187,221). An association with polydactyly is particularly common (11,13,187,221), as is syndactyly of the hands and feet concurrently (69,139). Bilateral and unilateral cases of syndactyly occur with approximately equal frequency (13,69,80,116,139,187), although a preponderance of unilateral cases occasionally has been reported (11,115). Among unilateral cases, an excess of syndactyly on the left side has generally been found (69,115,116); however, one series with more on the right side has also been reported (13).

Syndactyly most commonly involves only two digits on the hand or foot, but may involve three, four, or even all five digits (11,13,69,115,116). It occurs predominantly in the central rather than marginal digits (69,80,114,115). Among the central digits, syndactyly most frequently affects the middle and ring fingers (11,13,69, 80,114,139,187) and the second and third toes (13,80,187).

Estimated prevalence rates of syndactyly at birth generally range from about 0.3 per 1000 to 2 per 1000 (13,80,114,115,187). In one study (13) prevalence rates reported separately for the hands and feet were 1.4 per 1000 and 2.2 per 1000, respectively. Males are affected about twice as frequently as females (11,13,50,69,70,114,115,116,139). Prevalence rates are much higher in whites than in blacks, with estimates of the risk differential ranging from threefold to tenfold (39,50,92,187).

From 18 to 40 percent of cases have a family history of syndactyly (13,50,69,115,116), and while heredity is undoubtedly involved in the etiology, the mode of inheritance is not at all clear. Within many families the pattern of inheritance has appeared to be autosomal dominant with reduced penetrance (69,80,208,221,227). However, other families do not follow this pattern, and recessive genes, mutant genes, polygenic inheritance, and environmental factors have been postulated as causes (221). Although several exogenous factors, such as in utero exposure to infections, drugs, irradiation, and local mechanical stresses, have been suggested as etiologic agents (69), none has been established as a risk factor with any degree of certainty.

Both the endogenous and exogenous factors that may be involved in the etiology are thought to affect embryonic development during the fifth to eighth weeks of embryonic life, when adjacent digits are differentiating (69,70,80,114). An alternative mechanism, whereby syndactyly occurs as a readhesion of adjacent digits as a result of close contact between raw surfaces, has also been suggested (69,70) but is not widely accepted.

Polydactyly

In polydactyly there are more than five digits on a hand or foot. Three major types of polydactyly have been described (11,80): (1) an extra fleshy mass that does not adhere to the skeleton and which usually has no bones, cartilage, muscles, or tendons, (2) duplication of a normal digit that contains typical bone structure and that is attached to either an enlarged bifurcated metacarpal or metatarsal, (3) an extra digit associated with its own extra metacarpal or metatarsal bone; this is the most rare.

Polydactyly, which may be corrected surgically by removing the extra digit, can occur as an isolated malformation, in conjunction with other anomalies, or as part of several syndromes such as the Laurence-Moon-Biedl-Bardet syndrome (mental retardation, obesity, genital dysmorphism, and retinal pigmentosa) and the Ellis-van Creveld syndrome (dwarfism and cardiac anomalies) (187). It can occur both unilaterally and bilaterally, although the relative frequency of each is not agreed upon (11,13,194). Based on the known time sequence of normal embryonic and fetal development, Kelikian (114) has postulated that whatever the etiologic agents are, they are likely to have their effect during the sixth week of embryonic life.

Although any of the five digits may be involved, polydactyly tends to involve the marginal digits (11,13,80,89,194,218,221). Flatt (80) estimated that polydactyly of the small finger is eight times more common than all other forms. However, it appears that while small finger duplication is most common among blacks (194), the thumb is most often affected in white or Oriental cases (80,89,218,221). Index finger involvement is least common (80,218), although Burman (25) suggested that there may be misclassification of cases between thumb and index finger duplications.

Reported prevalence rates among livebirths in the United States have ranged from 0.5 per 1000 in Utah (221) to 2.9 per 1000 in Brooklyn (192). Rates within this same range have been noted in Japan (151,160) and in Southern Chinese prisoners (89), while somewhat higher rates of 3.7 per 1000 for the hands and 0.8 per 1000 for the feet have been observed in Sweden. In Uganda, over one percent of liveborn infants are reported to be affected with polydactyly (194).

Much of this variation in reported prevalence rates is due to the different racial compositions of the populations studied. In the United States polydactyly occurs at least nine times more frequently in blacks than in whites (39,81,92,192), with small finger duplications, in particular, being ten times more common in blacks than in whites (80,208). Rates among Orientals and Puerto Ricans appear to be intermediate between those of blacks and whites (80,92,160). Males and females have approximately equal rates, with some studies finding a slight excess among females (13,221) and others reporting an excess in males (114).

Familial aggregation of polydactyly has been reported repeatedly. Analysis of some pedigrees has suggested autosomal dominant inheritance in certain families (13,80,109,114,187,221,227), while pedigrees from other families as well as the occurrence of sporadic cases without apparent history of polydactyly or other "dactyly" anomalies suggests the existence of other modes of transmission or as yet unknown nongenetic factors (13,80,221).

Limb Reduction Deformities

A limb reduction deformity, sometimes called a congenital amputation, is total or partial absence of an arm, leg, finger, or toe in a newborn. Incomplete or rudimentary extremities occur more frequently than complete absence of limbs (163), and deformities more often affect the arms than the legs (126,163).

Most limb defects occur during the embryonic phase of differentiation, and the various clinical types of limb reduction are felt to represent varying degrees of destruction within the organization of the limb mesenchyme. The particular type of deformity that occurs is believed to be determined at least in part by the stage of development of the particular part of a bone at the time the etiologic agent is operative (206,207). General agreement does not exist as to whether reduction deformities as a group are associated with other congenital anomalies, including other limb anomalies (92,126,182).

Reported prevalence rates of limb reduction deformities at birth are influenced considerably by such factors as the diagnostic criteria used and by whether stillbirths and fetal death are included along with livebirths in the denominator of the prevalence rate. Unfortunately, in some studies it is not clear what conditions are included as reduction deformities or what types of births are included in the denominators of rates. The prevalence rates reported from the Collaborative Perinatal Project (92) were

0.6 per 1000 livebirths and stillbirths if only absence of a limb or part of a limb is included and 1.6 per 1000 if hypoplasia of a limb or part of a limb is counted as well. Data on "reduction deformities" from the Centers for Disease Control Birth Defects Monitoring Program (34) show rates of around 0.4 per 1000 livebirths and stillbirths for the United States (see Table 2-1). No marked differences in prevalence rates by geographic area have been reported. A 33 percent increase in prevalence rates using birth records in New York State from 1963 to 1973 has been noted, with the rate reaching 0.24 per 1000 in 1973 (108).

Male and female infants are affected with approximately equal frequency (108,182). Although slightly higher prevalence rates in Puerto Ricans (0.9 per 1000) and in whites (0.7 per 1000) than in blacks (0.5 per 1000) have been suggested (92), these rates are based on relatively small numbers of cases, particularly for the Puerto Ricans. In Edinburgh (182) no association of reduction deformities with socioeconomic status was found, whereas in New York State (108) both mothers and fathers of cases had slightly lower educational levels than did control parents. The former study (182) showed an excess of illegitimate children among cases, while the latter excluded illegitimate births.

The risk factor for limb reduction deformities that is best documented is use of thalidomide during pregnancy. Thalidomide is most strongly associated with phocomelia, a deformity characterized by absence of the proximal portion of a limb or limbs, with the hands or feet attached to the trunk by a single small irregularly shaped bone. Complete absence of a limb or limbs also was frequently associated with thalidomide, with all four limbs commonly involved (100). A "thalidomide syndrome" has been described, consisting of bilateral phocomelia and facial and internal malformations. Most of these cases had abnormalities of the long bones of the arms, and about half had lower limb involvement as well (206). Because phocomelia was so rare before the introduction of thalidomide, occurring in only about 1 per 75,000 births (206), the marked increase in the early 1960s in Europe was easily seen (100).

Other maternal factors associated with limb reduction deformities have been proposed but little is known with certainty; those suggested include young maternal age (182), hydramnios and oligamnios (182), maternal toxemia (182), twinning (108), and exposure to steroid hormones during early pregnancy, especially among male infants (108). Janerich et al. (108) have pointed out the possibility that women who report that they become pregnant while using oral contraceptives may have an underlying endocrine disorder that could itself predispose to limb reduction deformities in the offspring. An alternative hypothesis is that the oral contraceptive failures occur because of pharmacological inhibition by other concurrently used drugs, and that it is these drugs that cause the deformities (113).

Although it is felt that genetic factors may play a role in some types of reduction deformities, most investigators feel that the sporadic nature of these cases and the lack of recurrence within families suggest that environmental factors account for the majority of cases (126,134,182).

REFERENCES

1. Aarskog, D., Stoa, K. F., and Thorsen, T. 1966. "Urinary oestrogen excretion in newborn infants with congenital dysplasia of the hip joint." *Acta Paed. Scand.* 55:394–397.
2. Alberman, E. 1965. "The causes of congenital club foot." *Arch. Dis. Childhood* 40:548–554.
3. Andrèn, L. 1961. "Frequency and sex distribution of congenital dislocation of the hip among breech presentations." *Acta Orthop. Scand.* 31:152–155.
4. ———. 1962. "Pelvic instability in newborns with special reference to congenital dislocation of the hip and hormonal factors. A roentgenologic study." *Acta Radiol. Suppl.* 212:1–66.
5. Anonymous. 1971. "Epidemics of anencephaly and spina bifida." *Lancet* 1:689–690.
6. Archer, V. E. 1979. "Anencephalus, drinking water, geomagnetism and cosmic radiation." *Amer. J. Epid.* 109:88–97.
7. Aston, J. N. 1967. *A Short Textbook of Orthopaedics and Traumatology.* Philadelphia: Lippincott.
8. Atlas, S., Menacho, L. C. S., and Ures, S. 1980. "Some new aspects in the pathology of clubfoot." *Clin. Orthop.* 149:224–228.
9. Baird, D. 1974. "Epidemiology of congenital malformations of the central nervous system in (a) Aberdeen and (b) Scotland." *J. Biosoc. Sci.* 6:113–137.
10. Barlow, T. G. 1962. "Early diagnosis and treatment of congenital dislocation of the hip." *J. Bone Jt. Surg. (Brit.)* 44:292–301.
11. Barsky, A. J. 1951. "Congenital anomalies of the hand." *J. Bone Jt. Surg. (Amer.)* 33:35–64.
12. Beals, R. K. 1978. "Clubfoot in the Maori: A genetic study of fifty kindreds." *New Zeal. Med. J.* 88:144–146.
13. Beckman, L., and Widlund, L. 1962. "On the inheritance of poly- and syndactylies in man." *Acta Genet. Med. Gem* 11:43–54.
14. Ben-Menachem, Y., and Butler, J. 1974. "Arteriography of the foot in congenital deformities." *J. Bone Jt. Surg. (Amer.)* 56:1625–1630.
15. Berkman, L., Lempeig, R., and Nordstrom, M. 1977. "Congenital dislocation of the hip in Northern Sweden." *Clin. Genet.* 11:151–153.
16. Bick, E. M. 1960. "Congenital deformities of the musculoskeletal system noted in the newborn." *Amer. J. Dis. Child* 100:861–868.
17. Biggar, R. J., Mortimer, E. A., Jr., and Haughie, G. E. 1976. "Descriptive epidemiology of neural tube defects, Rochester, New York, 1918–1938." *Amer. J. Epid.* 104:22–27.

18. ———et al. 1976. "The relationship of supplemental iodine to neural tube defects in Rochester, New York, 1924–1932." *Amer. J. Epid.* 104:28–33.

19. Bjerkedal, T., and Bakketeig, L. S. 1975. "Surveillance of congenital malformations and other conditions of the newborn." *Int. J. Epid.* 4:31–36.

20. ———. 1974. "Congenital dislocation of the hip in Norway. I. Late diagnosis CDH." *Acta Orthop. Scand. Suppl.* 157:1–20.

21. ———. 1976. "Congenital dislocation of the hip in Norway. A clinical-epidemiological study." *J. Oslo City Hosp.* 26:79–90.

22. Bjonness, T. 1975. "Congenital clubfoot. A follow-up of 95 persons treated in Sweden from 1940–1945 with special reference to their social adaption and subjective symptoms from the foot." *Acta Orthop. Scand.* 46:848–856.

23. Bracken, M. B., Holford, T. R., White, C., and Kelsey, J. L. 1978. "Role of oral contraception in congenital malformations of offspring." *Int. J. Epid.* 7:309–317.

24. Brock, D. J. H., and Scrimgeour, J. B. 1974. "Alpha-feto protein in the prenatal diagnosis of C.N.S. malformations." *Lancet* 1:569.

25. Burman, M. 1972. "Note on duplications of the index finger." *J. Bone Jt. Surg. (Amer.)* 54:884.

26. Caffey, J., Ames, R., Silverman, W. A., Ryder, C. T., and Hough, G. 1956. "Contradiction of the congenital dysplasia—predislocation hypothesis of congenital dislocation of the hip through a study of normal variation in acetabular angles at successive periods in infancy." *Pediatrics* 17:632–641.

27. Carter, C. O. 1963. "Genetic factors in congenital dislocation of the hip." *Proc. Roy. Soc. Med.* 56:803–804.

28. ———. 1969. "Spina bifida and anencephaly: A problem in genetic-environmental interaction." *J. Biosoc. Sci.* 1:71–83.

29. ———, David, P. A., and Lawrence, K. M. 1968. "A family study of major central nervous system malformations in South Wales." *J. Med. Genet.* 5:81–106.

30. ———, and Evans, K. 1973. "Children of adult survivors with spina bifida cystica." *Lancet* 2:924–926.

31. ———, and Evans, K. 1973. "Spina bifida and anencephalus in Greater London." *J. Med. Genet.* 10:209–234.

32. ———, and Wilkinson, J. 1964. "Persistent joint laxity and congenital dislocation of the hip." *J. Bone Jt. Surg. (Brit.)* 46:40–45.

33. Center for Disease Control. 1976. *Congenital Malformations Surveillance Report,* January–December, 1975. Center for Disease Control, Atlanta, Georgia.

34. ———. 1980. Birth Defects Monitoring Program. Congenital Malformation Cases and Incidence Rates. Unpublished data.

35. ———. 1979. *Congenital Malformations Surveillance Report* July 1977–June 1978. HEW Publication No. (CDC) 79-8362.

36. Charlton, P. J. 1966. "Seasonal variation in incidence of some congenital malformations in two Australian samples." *Med. J. Aust.* 18:833–835.

37. Chen, R. Weisman, S. L., Salama, R., and Klingberg, M. A. 1970. "Congenital dislocation of the hip (CDH) and seasonality: The gestational age of vulnerability to some seasonal factor." *Amer. J. of Epid.* 92:287–293.

38. Ching, G. H. S., Chung, C. S., and Nemechek, R. W. 1969. "Genetic and epidemiologic studies of clubfoot in Hawaii: Ascertainment of incidence." *Amer. J. Hum. Genet.* 21:566–580.

39. Chung, C. S., and Myrianthopoulos, N. C. 1968. "Racial and prenatal factors in major congenital malformations." *Amer. J. Human Genet.* 20:44–60.

40. ———, Nemechek, R. W., Larsen, I. J., and Ching, G. 1969. "Genetic and epidemiologic studies of clubfoot in Hawaii. Genetic and medical considerations." *Human Hered.* 19:321–342.

41. Clarke, C., Hobson, D., McKendrick, O. M., Rogers, S. C., and Sheppard, P. M. 1975. "Spina bifida and anencephaly: Miscarriage as a possible cause." *Brit. Med. J.* 2:743–746.

42. ———, McKendrick, O. M., and Sheppard, P. M. 1973. "Spina bifida and potatoes." *Brit. Med. J.* 3:251–254.

43. Coleman, S. S. 1956. "Diagnosis of congenital dysplasia of the hip in the newborn." *J. Amer. Med. Ass.* 162:548–554.

44. Collmann, R. D., and Stoller, A. 1968. "The occurrence of anencephalus in the state of Victoria, Australia." *J. Ment. Defic. Res.* 12:22–35.

45. Creasy, M. R., and Alberman, E. D. 1976. "Congenital malformations of the central nervous system in spontaneous abortion." *J. Med. Genet.* 13:9–16.

46. Crelin, E. S. 1976. "An experimental study of hip stability in human newborn cadavers." *Yale J. Biol. Med.* 49:109–121.

47. Cyvin, K. B. 1977. "Congenital dislocation of the hip joint." *Acta Paediatr. Scand. Suppl.* 263:1–67.

48. Czeizel, A., Szentpetery, J., and Kellerman, M. 1974. "Incidence of congenital dislocation of the hip in Hungary." *Brit. J. Prev. Soc. Med.* 28:265–267.

49. ———, Tusnady, G., Vaczo, G., and Vizkelety, T. 1975. "The mechanisms of genetic predisposition in congenital dislocation of the hip." *J. Med. Genet.* 12:121–124.

50. Davis, J. S., and German, W. J. 1930. "Syndactylism." *Arch. Surg.* 21:32–75.

51. Dunn, P. 1974. "Congenital postural deformities: Further perinatal associations." *Proc. Roy. Soc. Med.* 67:1174–1178.

52. Dykes, R. G. 1975. "Congenital dislocation of the hip in Southland." *New Zeal. Med. J.* 81:467–470.

53. Edelstein, J. 1966. "Congenital dislocation of the hip in the Bantu." In proceedings and reports of universities, colleges, councils, and associations. *J. Bone Jt. Surg. (Brit.)* 48:397.

54. Edwards, J. H. 1958. "Congenital malformations of the central nervous system in Scotland." *Brit. J. Prev. Soc. Med.* 12:115–130.

55. ———. 1961. "Seasonal incidence of congenital disease in Birmingham." *Ann. Hum. Genet.* 25:89–93.

56. Elliot, J. K. 1961. "Clubfoot in the Polynesian." *J. Bone Jt. Surg. (Brit.)* 43:190.

57. Elwood, J. H. 1970. "Anencephalus in Belfast. Incidence, secular and seasonal variations 1950–1966." *Brit. J. Prev. Med.* 24:78–88.

58. ———. 1973. "Epidemics of anencephalus and spina bifida in Ireland since 1900." *Int. J. Epid.* 2:171–175.

59. ———, and Nevin, N. C. 1973. "Factors associated with anencephalus and spina bifida in Belfast." *Brit. J. Prev. Soc. Med.* 27:73–80.

60. Elwood, J. M. 1973. "Anencephaly and potato blight in Eastern Canada." *Lancet* 1:769.

61. ———. 1974. "Anencephalus in Canada 1943–1970." *Amer. J. Epid.* 100:288–296.

62. ———. 1976. "Anencephalus and spina bifida in North America." In *Birth Defects: Risks and Consequences*. S. Kelley et al., eds. New York: Academic Press, pp. 3–20.

63. ———. 1977. "Anencephalus and drinking water composition." *Amer. J. Epid.* 105:460–467.

64. ———. 1979. Comments on "Anencephalus, drinking water, geomagnetism, and cosmic radiation." *Amer. J. Epid.* 109:98–102.

65. ———, and Elwood, J. H. 1980. *Epidemiology of Anencephalus and Spina Bifida*. Oxford: Oxford University Press.

66. ———, and McBride, M. L. 1979. "Contrasting effects of maternal fertility and

birth rank on the occurrence of neural tube defects." *J. Epid. Comm. Hlth.* 33:78–83.

67. ———, Raman, S., and Mousseau, G. 1978. "Reproductive history in the mothers of anencephalics." *J. Chron. Dis.* 31:473–481.

68. Emanuel, I., and Sever, L. E. 1973. "Questions concerning the possible association of potatoes and neural tube defects, and an alternative hypothesis relating to maternal growth and development." *Teratology* 8:325–332.

69. Emmet, A. J. J. 1963. "Syndactyly of the hand: A review of 60 cases." *Brit. J. Plast. Surg.* 16:357–375.

70. Entin, M. A. 1978. "Congenital syndactyly: A reappraisal." *Can. J. Surg.* 21:360–364.

71. Epstein, B. S. 1976. *The Spine. A Radiological Text and Atlas.* Philadelphia: Lea and Febiger.

72. Fedrick, J. 1970. "Anencephalus and the local water supply." *Nature* 227:176–177.

73. ———. 1974. "Anencephalus and maternal tea drinking: Evidence for a positive association." *Proc. Roy. Soc. Med.* 67:356–360.

74. ———. 1976. "Anencephalus in Scotland 1961–72." *Brit. J. Prev. Soc. Med.* 30:132–137.

75. ———, and Adelstein, P. 1976. "Area differences in the incidence of neural tube defect and the rate of spontaneous abortion." *Brit. J. Prev. Soc. Med.* 30:32–35.

76. Field, B. 1978. "Neural tube defects in New South Wales, Australia." *J. Med. Genet.* 15:329–338.

77. ———, and Kerr,C. 1976. "Aetiology of anencephaly and spina bifida." *Brit. Med. J.* 2:107.

78. Fielding, D. W., and Smithells, R. W. 1971. "Anencephalus and water hardness in south-west Lancashire." *Brit. J. Prev. Soc. Med.* 25:217–219.

79. Finlay, H. V. L., Maudsley, R. H., and Busfield, P. I. 1967. "Dislocatable hip and dislocated hip in the newborn infant." *Brit. Med. J.* 4:377–381.

80. Flatt, A. E. 1977. *The Care of Congenital Hand Anomalies.* St. Louis: The C. V. Mosby Co.

81. Frazier, T. M. 1960. "A note on race-specific congenital malformation rates." *Amer. J. Obstet. Gynec.* 80:184–185.

82. Gardiner, A., Clarke, C., Cowen, J., Finn, R., and McKendrick, O. M. 1978. "Spontaneous abortion and fetal abnormality in subsequent pregnancy." *Brit. Med. J.* 2:1016–1018.

83. Gardner, W. J., and Breuer, A. C. 1980. "Anomalies of heart, spleen, kidneys, gut, and limbs may result from an overdistended neural tube: A hypothesis." *Pediatrics* 85:508–514.

84. Getz, B. 1955. "The hip joint in Lapps." *Acta Orthop. Scand. Suppl.* 28:1–81.

85. Gittelsohn, A. M., and Milham, S. 1962. "Declining incidence of central nervous system anomalies in New York State." *Brit. J. Prev. Soc. Med.* 16:153–158.

86. Golding, J. S. R. 1970. "Discussion." In proceedings and reports of universities, colleges, councils and associations. *J. Bone Jt. Surg. (Brit.)* 52:785.

87. Granroth, G., Hakama, M., and Saxen, L. 1977. "Defects of the central nervous system in Finland: I." *Brit. J. Prev. Soc. Med.* 31:164–170.

88. Halperin, L. R., and Wilroy, R. S., Jr. 1978. "Maternal hyperthermia and neural-tube defects." *Lancet* 2:212–213.

89. Handforth, J. R. 1950. "Polydactylism of the hand in Southern Chinese." *Anat. Rec.* 106:119–125.

90. Harlap, S., and Davies, A. M. 1978. The Pill and Births: The Jerusalem Study Final Report.

91. ———, Davies, A. M., Haber, M., Rossman, H., Prywes, R., and Samueloff, N.

1971. "Congenital malformations in the Jerusalem perinatal study. An overview with special reference to maternal origin." *Israeli J. Med. Sci.* 7:1520–1528.

92. Heinonen, O. P., Slone, D., and Shapiro, S. 1977. *Birth Defects and Drugs in Pregnancy.* Littleton, Mass.: Publishing Sciences Group.

93. Hewitt, D. 1963. "Geographical variations in the mortality attributed to spina bifida and other congenital malformations." *Brit. J. Prev. Soc. Med.* 17:13–22.

94. Hodgson, A. R. 1961. "Congenital dislocation of the hip." *Brit. Med. J.* 2:647.

95. Horowitz, I., and McDonald, A. D. 1969. "Anencephaly and spina bifida in the province of Quebec." *Can. Med. Assoc. J.* 100:748–755.

96. Howie, R. N., and Phillips, L. I. 1970. "Congenital malformations in the newborn: A survey at the National Women's Hospital, 1964–67." *New Zeal. Med. J.* 71:65–71.

97. Idelberger, K. 1939. "Die ergebnisse der zwillingforschung beim angborenen Klumpfuss." *Verhandlungen der Deutschen Orthopadischen Gesellschaft* 33:272–275.

98. Ingalls, T. H., Pugh, T. F., and MacMahon, B. 1954. "Incidence of anencephalus, spina bifida, and hydrocephalus related to birth rank and maternal age." *Brit. J. Prev. Soc. Med.* 8:17–23.

99. Irani, R. N., and Sherman, M. S. 1963. "The pathological anatomy of idiopathic clubfoot." *J. Bone Jt. Surg. (Amer.)* 45:45–62.

100. James, J. I. P., and Lamb, D. W. 1963. "Congenital abnormalities of the limbs." *The Practitioner* 191:159–172.

101. James, W. H. 1978. "Birth ranks of spontaneous abortions in sibships of children affected by anencephaly or spina bifida." *Brit. Med. J.* 1:72–73.

102. Janerich, D. T. 1972. "Anencephaly and maternal age." *Amer. J. Epid.* 95:319–326.

103. ———. 1972. "Maternal age and spina bifida: Longitudinal versus cross-sectional analysis." *Amer. J. Epid.* 96:389–395.

104. ———. 1973. "Epidemic waves in the prevalence of anencephaly and spina bifida in New York State." *Teratology* 8:253–256.

105. ———. 1974. "Endocrine dysfunction and anencephaly and spina bifida: An epidemiologic hypothesis." *Amer. J. Epid.* 99:1–7.

106. ———. 1975. "Female excess in anencephaly and spina bifida: Possible gestational influences." *Amer. J. Epid.* 101:70–76.

107. ———, and Piper, J. 1978. "Shifting genetic patterns of anencephaly and spina bifida." *J. Med. Genet.* 15:101–105.

108. ———, Piper, J., and Glebatis, D. 1974. "Oral contraceptives and congenital limb reduction defects." *New Engl. J. Med.* 291:697–700.

109. Johnston, O., and Davis, P. W. 1953. "On the inheritance of hand and foot anomalies in 6 families." *Amer. J. Hum. Genet.* 8:356–372.

110. Jones, D. H. 1965. "The early diagnosis of congenital dislocation of the hip joint." *Brit. J. Clin. Pract.* 19:443–449.

111. Kallen, B., and Winberg, J. 1968. "A Swedish register of congenital malformations. Experience with continuous registration during two years with special reference to multiple malformations." *Pediatrics* 41:765–776.

112. Katz, J. F., and Challenor, Y. B. 1974. "Childhood orthopedic syndromes." In *The Child with Disabling Illness.* J. A. Downey and N. L. Low, eds. Philadelphia: Saunders.

113. Kay, C. R. 1975. "Oral contraceptives and congenital limb-reduction defects." *New Engl. J. Med.,* Letter to Editor. 292:267–268.

114. Kelikian, H. 1974. *Congenital Deformities of the Hand and Forearm.* Philadelphia: Saunders.

115. Kettelkamp, D. B., and Flatt, A. E. 1961. "An evaluation of syndactylia repair." *Surg. Gynec. and Obst.* 113:471–478.
116. Kite, J. H. 1958. "Congenital syndactyly of the fingers." *Southern Med. J.* 51:160–164.
117. ———. 1964. *The Clubfoot.* New York: Grune and Stratton.
118. Klingberg, M. A., Chen, R., Chemke, J., and Levin, S. 1976. "Rising rates of congenital dislocation of the hip." *Lancet* 1:298.
119. ———, et al. 1976. "Rising rates of congenital dislocation of the hip." *Lancet* 1:547.
120. Knox, E. G. 1970. "Fetus-fetus interaction—a model aetiology for anencephalus." *Dev. Med. Child Neurol.* 12:167–177.
121. ———. 1972. "Anencephalus and dietary intakes." *Brit. J. Prev. Soc. Med.* 26:219–223.
122. ———. 1974. "Diet and anencephalus." *Proc. Roy. Soc. Med.* 67:355–356.
123. ———. 1974. "Twins and neural tube defects." *Brit. J. Prev. Soc. Med.* 28:73–80.
124. Kraus, B. S., and Schwartzmann, J. R. 1957. "Congenital dislocation of the hip among the Fort Apache Indians." *J. Bone Jt. Surg. (Amer.)* 39:448–449.
125. Kuhr, M. D. 1977. "Neural-tube defects and mid-cycle abstinence: A test of the 'over-ripeness' hypothesis in man." *Develop. Med. Child. Neurol.* 19:589–592.
126. Lamy, M., and Maroteaux, P. 1969. "The genetic study of limb malformations." In *Limb Development and Deformity: Problems of Evaluation and Rehabilitation.* C. A. Swinyard, ed. Springfield, Ill.: Charles C Thomas.
127. Laurence, K. M. 1969. "The recurrence risk in spina bifida cystica and anencephaly." *Dev. Med. Child. Neurol. Suppl.* 20:23–30.
128. ———, and Roberts, C. J. 1977. "Spina bifida and anencephaly: Are miscarriages a possible cause?" *Brit. Med. J.* 2:361–362.
129. Leck, I. 1966. "Changes in the incidence of neural-tube defects." *Lancet* 2:791–793.
130. ———.1972, "The etiology of human malformations: Insights from epidemiology." *Teratology* 5:303-311.
131 ———. 1974. "Causation of neural tube defects: Clues from epidemiology." *Brit. Med. Bull.* 30:158–163.
132. ———. 1976. "Rising rates of congenital dislocation of the hip." *Lancet* 1:372.
133. ———. 1978. "Maternal hyperthermia and anencephaly." *Lancet* 1:671–672.
134. Lenz, W. 1980. "Genetics and limb deficiencies." *Clin. Orthop.* 148:9–17.
135. Lorber, J. 1965. "The family history of spina bifida cystica." *Pediatrics* 35:589–595.
136. Lowe, C. R. 1972. "Congenital malformations and the problem of their control." *Brit. Med. J.* 2:515–520.
137. ———, Roberts, C. J., and Lloyd, S. 1971. "Malformations of central nervous system and softness of local water supplies." *Brit. Med. J.* 2:357–361.
138. MacAusland, W. R., Jr., and Mayo, R. A. 1965. *Orthopedics.* Boston: Little, Brown, and Company.
139. MacCollum, D. W. 1940. "Webbed fingers." *Surg. Gynec. and Obst.* 71:782–789.
140. MacKenzie, J. S., and Houghton, M. 1974. "Influenza infections during pregnancy." *Bacteriol. Rev.* 38:356–370.
141. MacMahon, B., Pugh, T. F., and Ingalls, T. S. 1953. "Anencephalus, spina bifida and hydrocephalus: Incidence related to sex, race, and season of birth, and incidence in siblings." *Brit. J. Prev. Soc. Med.* 7:211–219.
142. ———, and Yen, S. 1971. "Unrecognised epidemic of anencephaly and spina bifida." *Lancet* 1:31–33.

143. ———, Yen, S., and Rothman, K. J. 1973. "Potato blight and neural-tube defects." *Lancet* 1:598–599.

144. Matsoukas, J. A. and Papathassion, B. T. 1970. "Maternal thyroid disorders and infantile clubfoot. Is there a relationship?" *Clin. Pediat.* 9:201–202.

145. McBride, M. L. 1979. "Sib risks of anencephaly and spina bifida in British Columbia." *Amer. J. Med. Genet.* 3:377–387.

146. McIntosh, R., Merritt, K. K., Richards, M. R., Samuels, M. H., and Bellows, M. T. 1954. "The incidence of congenital malformations: A study of 5964 pregnancies." *Pediatrics* 14:505–522.

147. McKeown, T., and Record, R. G. 1951. "Seasonal incidence of congenital malformations of the central nervous system." *Lancet* 1:192–196.

148. Medalie, J. H. Makin, M., Alkalay, E., Yofe, J., Cochari, Z., and Ehrlich, D. 1966. "Congenital dislocation of the hip, a clinical-epidemiological study, Jerusalem 1954–1960: I. Retrospective incidence study." *Israeli J. Med. Sci.* 2:212–217.

149. Miller, M., Vowles, M., Evans, K., and Carter, C. 1971. "Hormonal pregnancy tests and neural tube malformations." *Nature* 233:495–496.

150. Miller, P., Smith, D., and Shepard, T. H. 1978. "Maternal hyperthermia as a possible cause of anencephaly." *Lancet* 1:519–521.

151. Mitani, S. 1954. "Malformations of the newborn infants." *J. Jap. Obstet. Gynaec. Soc.* 1:301.

152. Mortimer, E. A. 1980. "The puzzling epidemiology of neural tube defects." *Pediatrics* 65:636–638.

153. Muller, G. M. and Seddon, H. J. 1953. "Late results of the treatment of congenital dislocation of the hip." *J. Bone Jt. Surg. (Brit.)* 35:342–362.

154. Naderi, S. 1975. "Smallpox vaccination during pregnancy." *Obstet. Gynec.* 46:223–226.

155. Naggan, L. 1969. "The recent decline in prevalence of anencephaly and spina bifida." *Amer. J. Epid.* 89:154–160.

156. ———. 1971. "Anencephaly and spina bifida in Israel." *Pediatrics* 47:577–586.

157. ———, and MacMahon, B. 1967. "Ethnic differences in the prevalence of anencephaly and spina bifida in Boston, Massachusetts." *N. Engl. J. Med.* 277:1119–1123.

158. Nakano, K. K. 1973. "Anencephaly: A review." *Dev. Med. Child. Neurol.* 15:383–400.

159. Nance, W. W. 1969. "Anencephaly and spina bifida: A possible example of cytoplasmic inheritance in man." *Nature* 224:373–375.

160. Neel, J. V. 1958. "A study of major congenital defects in Japanese infants." *Amer. J. Hum. Genet.* 10:398–445.

161. Niclasen, S. D. 1978. "Family studies of relation between Perthes' disease and congenital dislocation of the hip." *J. Med. Genet.* 15:296–299.

162. Nishimura, H. 1970. "Incidence of malformations in abortions." In *Congenital Malformations, Proceedings of the Third International Conference*. F. C. Fraser, and V. A. McKusick, eds. Amsterdam: Excerpta Medica Foundation, pp. 275–283.

163. ———, and Okamoto, N. 1976. *Sequential Atlas of Human Congenital Malformations*. Baltimore: University Park Press.

164. Oakley, G. P., Flynt, J. W., and Falk, A. 1973. "Hormonal pregnancy tests and congenital malformations." *Lancet* 2:256–257.

165. Palmer, R. M. 1964. "The genetics of talipes equinovarus." *J. Bone Jt. Surg. (Amer.)* 46:542–556.

166. ———, Conneally, P. M., and Yu, P. 1974. "Studies of the inheritance of idiopathic talipes equinovarus." *Orthop. Clin. N. Am.* 5:99–108.

167. Phillips, L. J. 1968. "Congenital dislocation of the hip in the newborn: A survey at National Women's Hospital 1954–1958." *N. Zeal. Med. J.* 68:103–108.

168. Rabin, D. L., Barnett, C. R., Arnold, W. D., Freiberger, R. H., and Brooks, G. 1965. "Untreated congenital dislocation of the hip—A study of the epidemiology, natural history, and social aspects of the disease in a Navajo population." *Amer. J. Pub. Health* 55 Suppl.:1–44

169. Ralis, Z., and McKibbin, B. 1973. "Changes in the shape of the human hip joint during its development and their relation to its stability." *J. Bone Jt. Surg. (Brit.)* 55:780–785.

170. Record, R. C. 1961. "Anencephalus in Scotland." *Brit. J. Prev. Soc. Med.* 15:93–105.

171. ———, and Edwards, J. H. 1958. "Environmental influences related to the aetiology of congenital dislocation of the hip." *Brit. J. Prev. Soc. Med.* 12:8–22.

172. ———, and McKeown, T. 1949. "Congenital malformations of the central nervous system. I. A survey of 930 cases." *Brit. J. Soc. Med.* 3:183–219.

173. Reimann, I. 1967. *Congenital Idiopathic Clubfoot.* Copenhagen: Munksgaard.

174. Renwick, J. H. 1972. "Hypothesis: Anencephaly and spina bifida are usually preventable by the avoidance of a specific but unidentified substance present in certain potato tubers." *Brit. J. Prev. Soc. Med.* 26:67–88.

175. ———. 1973. "Prevention of anencephaly and spina bifida in man." *Teratology* 8:321–323.

176. Richards, I. D. 1969. "Congenital malformations and environmental influences in pregnancy." *Brit. J. Prev. Soc. Med.* 23:218–225.

177. Riser, W. H. 1975. "The dog as a model for the study of hip dysplasia. Growth, form, and development of the normal and dysplastic hip joint." *Vet. Pathol.* 12:234–334.

178. Roberts, C. J., and Lloyd, S. 1973. "Area differences in spontaneous abortion rates in South Wales and their relation to neural tube defect and incidence." *Brit. Med. J.* 4:20–22.

179. ———, and Lowe, C. R. 1975. "Where have all the conceptions gone?" *Lancet* 1:498–499.

180. ———, Revington, C. J., and Lloyd, S. 1973. "Potato cultivation and storage in South Wales and its relation to neural tube malformation prevalence." *Brit. J. Prev. Soc. Med.* 27:214–216.

181. Robinson, G. W. 1968. "Birth characteristics of children with congenital dislocation of the hip." *Amer. J. Epid.* 87:275–284.

182. Rogala, E. J., Wynne-Davies, R., Littlejohn, A., and Gormley, J. 1974. "Congenital limb anomalies: Frequency and aetiological factors." *J. Med. Genet.* 11:221–233.

183. Rogers, S. C., and Morris, M. 1971. "Infant mortality from spina bifida, congenital hydrocephalus, monstrosity, and congenital diseases of the cardiovascular system in England and Wales." *Ann. Hum. Genet.* 34:295–305.

184. ——— and Morris, M. 1973. "Anencephalus: A changing sex ratio." *Brit. J. Prev. Soc. Med.* 27:81–84.

185. ———, and Weatherall, J. A. C. 1976. *Anencephalus, spina bifida and congenital hydrocephalus: England and Wales, 1964–1972.* London: HM Stationery Office.

186. Royal College of General Practitioners. 1976. "The outcome of pregnancy in former oral contraceptive users." *Brit. J. Obstet. Gynaecol.* 83:608–616.

187. Ruby, L., and Goldberg, M. J. 1976. "Syndactyly and polydactyly." *Orthop. Clin. N. Amer.* 7:361–374.

188. St. Leger, A. S., and Elwood, P. C. 1980. "Neural tube malformations and trace elements in water." *J. Epid. Comm. Hlth.* 34:186–187.

189. Scrimgeour, J. B., and Cockburn, F. 1979. "Congenital abnormalities." *Lancet* 2:1349–1352.

190. Sever, L. E. 1978. "Epidemiologic aspects of neural tube defects." In *Prevention of Neural Tube Defects,* UCLA Forum in Medical Sciences, No. 21, pp. 75–89.

191. ———, and Emanuel, I. 1973. "Is there a connection between maternal zinc deficiency and congenital malformations of the central nervous system in man?" *Teratology* 7:117–118.

192. Shapiro, R. N., Eddy, W., Fitzgibbon, J., and O'Brien, G. 1958."The incidence of congenital anomalies discovered in the neonatal period." *Amer. J. Surg.* 96:396–400.

193. Siemiatycki, J., and McDonald, A. D. 1972. "Neural tube defects in Quebec. A search for evidence of 'clustering' in time and place." *Brit. J. Prev. Soc. Med.* 26:10–14.

194. Simpkiss, M., and Lowe, A. 1961. "Congenital abnormalities in the African newborn." *Arch. Dis. Child* 36:404–406.

195. Singer, H. A., Nelson, M. M., and Beighton, P. H. 1978. "Spina bifida and anencephaly in the Cape." *S. Afr. Med. J.* 53:626–630.

196. Smaill, G. B. 1968. "Congenital dislocation of the hip in the newborn." *J. Bone Jt. Surg. (Brit.)* 50:525–536.

197. Smith, C., Watt, M., Boyd, A. E. W., and Holmes, J. C. 1973. "Anencephaly, spina bifida, and potato blight in the Edinburgh area." *Lancet* 1:269.

198. Smith, D. W., Clarren, S. K., and Harvey, M. A. S. 1978. "Hyperthermia as a possible teratogenic agent." *J. Pediat.* 92:878–883.

199. Smithells, R. W., Sheppard, S., Schorah, C. J., Seller, M. J., Nevin, N. C., Harris, R., Read, A. P., and Fielding, D. W. 1980. "Possible prevention of neural tube defects by periconceptional vitamin supplementation." *Lancet* 1:339–340.

200. Spiers, P. S., Pietrzyk, J. J., Piper, J. M., and Glebatis, D. M. 1974. "Human potato consumption and neural tube malformation." *Teratology* 10:125–128.

201. Stevenson, A.C., Johnston, M. I. P., Stewart, M. I. P., and Golding, D. R. 1966. "Congenital malformations: A report of a study of series of consecutive births in 24 centres." *Bull. WHO* 34 (Suppl.), pp. 1–127.

202. Stewart, S. F. 1951. "Clubfoot: incidence, cause, and treatment." *J. Bone Jt. Surg. (Amer.)* 33:577–588.

203. Stocks, P. 1970. "Incidence of congenital malformations in the regions of England and Wales." *Brit. J. Prev. Soc. Med.* 24:66–77.

204. Strange, F. G. S. 1965. *The Hip.* London: Heinemann.

205. Stulberg, S. D., and Hanes, W. H. 1974. "Acetabular dysplasia and development of osteoarthritis of the hip." In *The Hip. Proceedings of the Second Open Scientific Meeting of the Hip Society.* W. H. Hanes, ed. St. Louis: The C. V. Mosby Co.

206. Sucheston, M. E., and Cannon, M. S. 1973. *Congenital Malformations: Case Studies In Developmental Anatomy.* Philadelphia: Davis.

207. Swanson, A. B. 1976. "A classification for congenital limb malformations." *J. Hand Surg.* 1:8–22.

208. Temtamy, S., and McKusick, V. A. 1969. "Synopsis of hand malformations with particular emphasis on genetic factors." *Birth Defects* 5:125–184.

209. Thieme, W. T., Wynne-Davis, R., Blair, H. A. F., Bell, E. T., and Loraine, J. A. 1968. "Clinical examination and urinary oestrogen assays in newborn children with congenital dislocation of the hip." *J. Bone Jt. Surg. (Brit.)* 50:546–550.

210. Trichopoulos, D., Desmond, L., Yen, S., and MacMahon, B. 1971. "A study of time-place clustering in anencephaly and spina bifida." *Amer. J. Epid.* 94:26–30.
211. Van Meerdervoort, H. F. P. 1974. "Congenital dislocation of the hip in Black patients." *S. Afr. Med. J.* 48:2436–2440.
212. Von Rosen, S. 1962. "Diagnosis and treatment of congenital dislocation of the hip joint in the new-born." *J. Bone Jt. Surg. (Brit.)* 44:284–291.
213. Walker, J. M. 1977. "Congenital hip disease in a Cree-Ojibwa population: a retrospective study." *Can. Med. Ass. J.* 116:501–504.
214. Wiberg, G. 1939. "Studies on dysplastic acetabular and congenital subluxation of the hip joint with special reference to the complication of osteoarthritis." *Acta Chir. Scand. Suppl.* 58.
215. ———. 1963. "Prime factors in the etiology of congenital dislocation of the hip." *J. Bone Jt. Surg. (Brit.)* 45:268–283.
216. Wiley, A. M. 1959. "An anatomical and experimental study of muscular growth." *J. Bone Jt. Surg. (Brit.)* 41:821–835.
217. Wilkinson, J. A. 1966. "Breech malposition and intrauterine dislocations." *Proc. Roy. Soc. Med.* 59:1106–1108.
218. Wood, V. E. 1970. "Duplication of the index finger." *J. Bone Jt. Surg. (Amer.)* 52:569–573.
219. Woolf, C. M., Koehn, J. H., and Coleman, S. S. 1968. "The congenital hip disease in Utah: The influence of genetic and nongenetic factors." *Amer. J. Hum. Genet.* 20:430–439.
220. ———, and Woolf, R. M. 1970. "A genetic study of polydactyly in Utah." *Amer. J. Hum. Genet.* 22:75–88.
221. ———, and Woolf, R. M. 1973. "A genetic study of syndactyly in Utah." *Soc. Biol.* 20:335–346.
222. Working Party on Amniocentesis. 1978. An assessment of the hazards of amniocentesis: Report to the Medical Research Council. *Brit. J. Obstet. Gyn.* 85:Suppl. 2.
223. Wynne-Davies, R. 1964. "Family studies and the cause of congenital clubfoot." *J. Bone Jt. Surg. (Brit.)* 46:445–463.
224. ———. 1965. "Family studies and aetiology of clubfoot." *J. Med. Genet.* 2:227–232.
225. ———. 1970. "Acetabular dysplasia and familial joint laxity: Two etiologic factors in congenital dislocation of the hip. A review of 589 patients and their families." *J. Bone Jt. Surg. (Brit.)* 52:704–716.
226. ———. 1970. "A family study of neonatal and late diagnosis of congenital dislocation of the hip." *J. Med. Genet.* 7:315–333.
227. ———. 1971. "Genetics and malformations of the hand." *Hand* 3:184–192.
228. ———. 1972. "Genetic and environmental factors in the etiology of talipes equinovarus." *Clin. Orthop.* 84:9–13.
229. Xilinas, M. E., and Largarde, D. 1975. "Congenital dislocation of the hip in Brittany." *Lancet* 1:863.
230. Yen, S., and MacMahon, B. 1968. "Genetics of anencephaly and spina bifida." *Lancet* 2:623–626.

3 Musculoskeletal Disorders of Childhood and Adolescence

Children and adolescents may be affected by a variety of musculoskeletal conditions. Most common are acute injuries, such as fractures, dislocations, sprains, and strains, which are discussed in Chapter 8. Each year more than 1 out of 10 individuals in the age group 6 to 16 years either seeks medical care or has activity restricted because of an injury (111). Fortunately, most of these injuries heal rapidly. In contrast, the diseases discussed in this chapter, and also juvenile rheumatoid arthritis (see Chapter 4), last over a period of a few years. Some residual deformity and early osteoarthrosis in the affected area may also occur unless prompt and effective treatment is administered. Of even greater severity are bone cancers (see Chapter 9), which are frequently fatal.

The disorders reviewed in this chapter are all related to growth, and a brief description of pertinent aspects of skeletal growth and maturation in childhood and adolescence may be helpful in understanding their pathogenesis.

The ends of long bones are originally cartilaginous, but as a child grows, osseous epiphyseal centers appear within the cartilage, the times of appearance of these centers varying from one bone to another. Legg-Calvé-Perthes disease, which is believed to be the result of inadequate blood supply to the growing epiphysis of the head of the femur, is the most commonly diagnosed of these osteochondroses of the "crushing" type, but other growing epiphyses also occasionally are affected. In Freiberg's disease, for instance, the head of the second or third metatarsal is involved.

The epiphysis of a long bone is separated from its shaft (the diaphysis) by a cartilage plate, called the epiphyseal plate. Growth in length of bone takes place in the area of the epiphyseal plate. When growth is completed, this plate disappears and bone is united to bone. During growth, the epiphysis of a bone occasionally becomes displaced off the diaphysis of the bone at the level of the epiphyseal plate. Again, the head of the femur is most frequently involved, and this disorder is called slipped capital femoral epiphysis.

Separate ossification centers appear at the ends of some long bones; these centers do not articulate directly with other bones, but may be situated at the point of attachment of muscles, for instance. Such a bony structure is called an apophysis. Disorders of developing apophyses may occur because of the strain resulting from the pulling of an attached tendon and are called "pulling" osteochondroses. These conditions are self-limiting, so that after the resolution of the strain, normal function is restored. The main symptom is localized pain. The most common of the pulling osteochondroses is Osgood-Schlatter's disease, or osteochondritis of the tibial tubercle. Sever's disease of the os calcis is another example of such a growth disorder.

Osteochondroses have been known to occur in main bony centers of other parts of the skeleton such as the tarsal navicular (Kohler's disease), the carpal lunate (Keinboch's disease), and the vertebral bodies (Calvé's disease). These occur very infrequently and will not be considered here.

Finally, growth disorders in the spine may result in abnormal curvature of the spine. Abnormal posterior curvature in adolescents is called kyphosis (or Scheuermann's disease), while abnormal lateral curvature with vertebral rotation is known as scoliosis. Although both disorders occur close to the time of adolescent growth spurt, in most cases the causes are not known. Scheuermann's disease is classified by some as a "crushing" type of osteochondrosis of the ring epiphysis of the vertebral body, but this is not universally accepted.

Legg-Calvé-Perthes disease, slipped epiphysis, and adolescent scoliosis have been studied to the extent that some knowledge of their epidemiologic characteristics currently exists. Very little, however, is known of the epidemiology of Osgood-Schlatter's disease and of Scheuermann's disease; the various etiologic hypotheses that have been formulated from clinical observations and animal experiments need to be followed up in human epidemiologic studies.

LEGG-CALVÉ-PERTHES DISEASE

This disease involves necrosis or degeneration of the ossification center of the head of the femur, followed by regeneration of normal bone and recal-

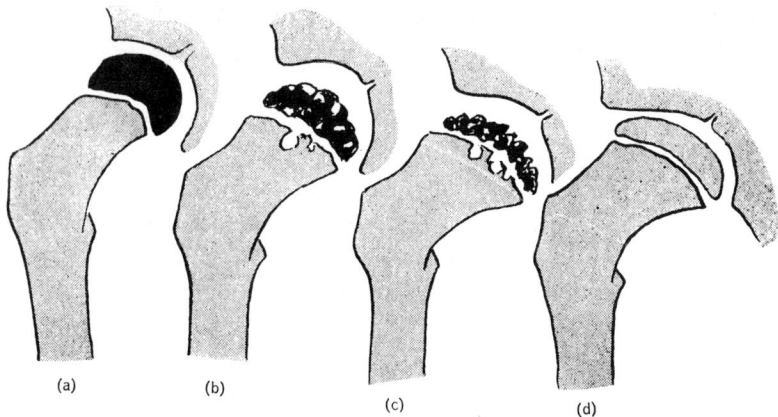

Figure 3-1 Serial changes in Legg-Calvé-Perthes disease.
Source: Aston (5).

cification (see Figure 3-1); the entire process tends to take from two to four years. It generally affects children of 4 to 8 years of age, and the usual symptoms are limp, muscle spasm, and pain. The lesion is thought to be a result of interference with the normal blood supply to this area. Experiments in puppies as well as autopsy observations suggest that the necrosis in Legg-Calvé-Perthes disease probably results from repeated ischemic episodes (72,77,89,103), although why these episodes should occur is not known. In children of around 4 to 7 years of age, the femoral epiphysis is nourished entirely by the lateral epiphyseal vessels that run along the femoral neck posterosuperiorly under the periosteum. This position is vulnerable to stress from compression and occlusion.

In Massachusetts, it was estimated that 1 in 740 males and 1 in 3700 females would be affected with Legg-Calvé-Perthes disease before the age of 15 years. The annual incidence rate in both sexes under age 15 was 5.7 per 100,000 (105). Similar incidence rates have been reported in Wessex, England (7), and in British Columbia, Canada (59), but higher rates of 11.1 per 100,000 and 7.6 per 100,000 have been found in Mersey and Trent, England, respectively (7). At least 1 in 10 affected children has the disease in both hips. In unilateral cases, the left and right hips are involved with approximately equal frequency (46,51,94,161).

Legg-Calvé-Perthes disease is most often seen in children from ages 4 to 8 years, although those up to the age of 15 years may be affected. It occurs in males four to five times more frequently than in females (see

Table 3-1 Incidence of Legg-Calvé-Perthes Disease by Age in White Residents of Massachusetts, 1964

Age (years)	Number of cases			Population	Incidence/100,000
	Males	Females	Totals		
<1	0	0	0	104,637	0.0
1	0	0	0	104,922	0.0
2	1	0	1	107,471	0.9
3	7	0	7	109,119	6.4
4	14	2	16	108,089	14.8
5	15	2	17	108,316	15.7
6	7	4	11	107,685	10.2
7	10	1	11	103,951	10.6
8	10	3	13	103,323	12.6
9	3	0	3	101,113	3.0
10	3	1	4	97,368	4.1
11	1	0	1	96,492	1.0
12	1	0	1	92,023	1.1
13	0	0	0	96,680	0.0
14	0	1	1	86,997	1.2
Totals	72	14	86	1,518,186	5.7

Source: Molloy and MacMahon (105). Reprinted by permission of the *New England Journal of Medicine,* 275: 988-990, 1966.

Table 3-1) (28,30,40,46,51,57,59,94,105,161); girls are on the average affected at a slightly younger age than boys (51,57). In both the United States and in Africa the disease has been found to occur infrequently in blacks (28,34,39,51,57,58,105). No overall difference in frequency was found by social class in one study (106), while another reported an excess of cases in lower social classes (161).

Some familial aggregation of cases in first-degree relatives has been reported (51,57,59,62,94,146,161). The extent to which this is attributable to genetic factors or to a common environment is not known. In any event, it is highly unlikely that a single gene is responsible for the occurrence of the disease, and most of the available evidence suggests that environmental factors are more important than hereditary ones (7,161).

Several investigators have found that children with Legg-Calvé-Perthes disease have slower-than-average skeletal maturation (see Figure 3-2) (28,30,51,65,101,105). Accordingly, these children tend to be short for their age (30,51,57,161). One study (24) has indicated that children with Legg-Calvé-Perthes disease have disproportionate growth in various

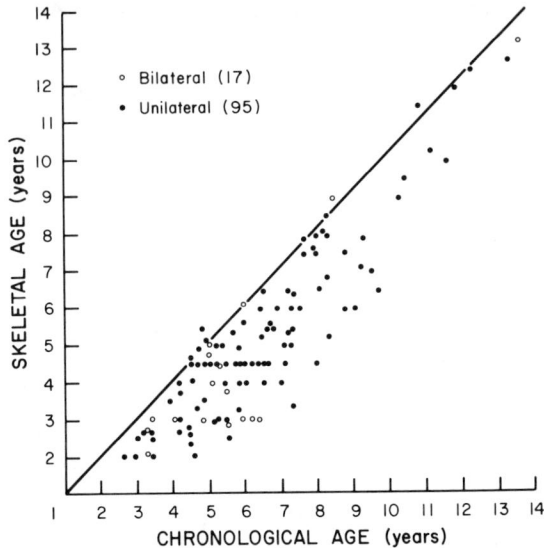

Figure 3-2   Skeletal age of males with Legg-Calvé-Perthes disease according to chronological age. Skeletal age was determined from wrist X-rays.

Source: Fisher (51).

parts of the body, suggesting that in affected children there is an abnormality of those mechanisms that determine the differential growth rates in various regions of the body. This finding requires further evaluation.

The evidence for a role of other suggested risk factors in Legg-Calvé-Perthes disease has been largely contradictory. For instance, conflicting results have been found in studies that have considered the associations of Legg-Calvé-Perthes disease with low birth weight (51,106,161) and with congenital abnormalities of the genitourinary tract and inguinal region (31,62,161). Such factors as older parental age, late birth order, breech presentation, other malposition, or version late in pregnancy have been reported by one group to occur with higher-than-expected frequency in children with this disease (161), but were not found by others (51,106). Trauma (28,40), synovitis (73), hypothyroidism (32,133), abnormal sensitivity to Vitamin D (105), and a generalized constitutional disorder (57,146) have been suggested as causal factors, but insufficient data have been presented to support these hypotheses. In fact, other investigators have not observed previous injuries and illnesses or hypothyroidism to be associated with Legg-Calvé-Perthes disease (46,51,106,161).

Thus, it has been established that boys, whites, and children undergoing slow skeletal maturation have an increased risk for Legg-Calvé-Perthes disease. Since whites tend to mature more slowly than blacks and boys more slowly than girls (55), hormonal factors may explain, at least in part, the higher incidence in whites and in boys. Experiments in dogs (96) also suggest an etiologic involvement of sex hormones. However, it is unknown why some children with slow maturation develop Legg-Calvé-Perthes disease while most do not. The hypothesis that disproportionate growth is etiologically involved merits further study. Also, careful epidemiologic testing of other existing hypotheses, such as those concerning perinatal and metabolic disorders, should be undertaken. Perhaps most of all, however, fresh ideas on etiology are needed.

OSGOOD-SCHLATTER'S DISEASE

This disease is an osteochondrosis of the tibial tubercle (the oblong elevation on the anterior surface of the upper end of the tibia to which the patellar ligament is attached). Although Osgood-Schlatter's disease is the most frequent of the osteochondroses (19), it is generally not serious, since the relatively small region in which it occurs is not involved in weight bearing. The disorder is characterized by pain and tenderness and by some enlargement of the tibial tubercle. The pain, which is localized in front of and below the knee, is increased in extension of the knee against resistance, since such extension leads to contracture of the patellar tendon on the tubercle. Recovery usually occurs spontaneously within several months.

Unlike Legg-Calvé-Perthes disease, Osgood-Schlatter's disease shows no evidence of primary vascular damage (43,114). Amputation and autopsy specimens from both dogs and humans have shown that the blood supply to the tibial tubercle is unimpaired. In addition, the radiographic patterns are unlike the sclerosis, collapse, porosis, and remodeling seen in Legg-Calvé-Perthes disease (114).

No figures are available on the prevalence or incidence of Osgood-Schlatter's disease in a defined population. It is diagnosed more frequently in males than in females (41), with the mean ages at onset of symptoms being about 13.5 years for boys and 11.5 years for girls (41,71). The earlier age at onset in girls corresponds to their earlier development of the apophysis of the tibial tuberosity. Unilateral cases occur about twice as frequently as bilateral cases (41). One investigator

(41) found no evidence of abnormal height-age and height-weight relationships, and no evidence of familial aggregation.

Very little is known of the etiology of this condition, but it is generally believed that direct trauma to and stress on the tibial tubercle are involved. Some patients do indicate that trauma preceded the onset of symptoms, and experiments in dogs have shown that trauma can produce lesions that are radiographically and histologically similar to the spontaneous pathological changes seen in Osgood-Schlatter's disease (42). However, fewer than half the patients with Osgood-Schlatter's disease report an injury prior to the development of symptoms (19,41), so that trauma does not appear to be a necessary cause.

Attention has also been paid to the possible etiologic role of pull from the patellar tendon on the tibial tubercle. Specifically, it has been hypothesized that injury to the lower end of the patellar tendon with resulting new bone formation is a cause (159). The possible importance of abnormal stress from the patellar tendon was also suggested by Willner (151), who found that all 78 cases of the disorder that he examined had an abnormal angle of insertion of the patellar tendon into the tibial tubercle. Adolescents may be particularly susceptible to the stress in this area for at least two reasons: (1) the very rapid growth during adolescence is a source of abnormal stress on the apophysis (47), and (2) prior to about the age of 18 years the center of ossification in the tibial tubercle is not united to the shaft; because strain from contraction of the quadriceps muscle is transmitted to the tubercle, it is in a vulnerable position until the apophysis is fused to the parent bone. Nevertheless, all of these hypotheses remain speculative.

SLIPPED CAPITAL FEMORAL EPIPHYSIS

This is primarily a disease of adolescents in which the epiphysis of the head of the femur is displaced backward and downward off the diaphysis (see Figure 3-3). The actual separation takes place through the layer of hypertrophied cartilage cells adjacent to the zone of calcifying cartilage of the epiphyseal plate (64,107,118). The usual symptoms are pain, stiffness, limp, and a limited range of motion of the hip joint. This disorder is closely related to the adolescent growth spurt and does not occur once the epiphysis is fused to the shaft of the femur.

Since slipped epiphysis is in general a painful and disabling condition for which the treatment almost always involves surgery, reasonable esti-

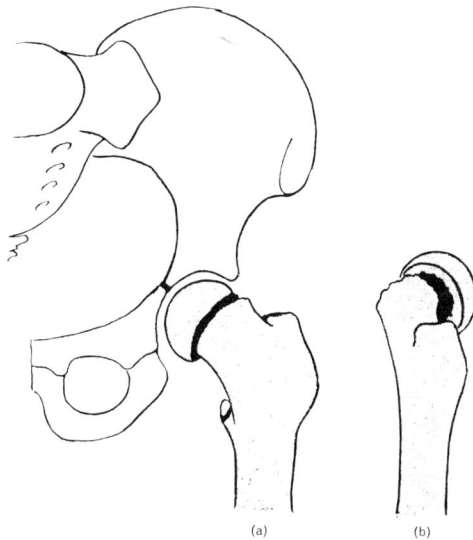

Figure 3-3   Slipped capital femoral epiphysis. (*a*) Anterior-posterior view. (*b*) Lateral view.

Source: Aston (5).

mates of incidence rates have been obtained by identifying new cases from records of hospitals serving defined geographic regions. The annual incidence of slipped epiphysis has been reported to be 3.4 per 100,000 in the population under 25 in Connecticut (83), 0.7 per 100,000 in New Mexico (86), and to range from 2 to 13 per 100,000 in the age group 7 to 17 years in Gothenburg, Sweden, over a period of several years (66). In Connecticut (86), it has been estimated that about 1 in 800 males and 1 in 2000 females will be diagnosed as having a slipped epiphysis before they reach the age of 25.

   Figure 3-4 shows that most cases occur between the ages of 10 and 17 years in males and 8 to 15 in females; the median age at diagnosis is 13 for males and 11 for females (78,83,86,90,107), the earlier age in females corresponding to their earlier onset of puberty. Occasionally a case is reported in a young child who has suffered severe trauma or who has some specific medical disorder such as tuberculosis or severe malnutrition (86,119). Also, a case may occur in an older person with delayed maturation (21,78,86). Males have been consistently found to be affected more frequently than females (78,83,86,90,107,139), although the ratio of males to females has varied from one geographic area to another. For

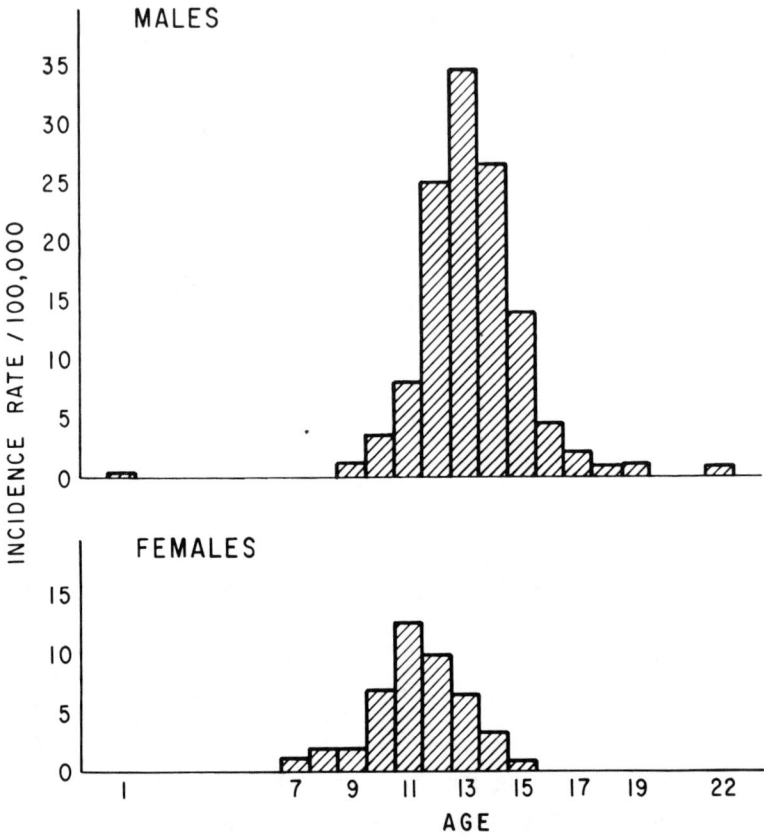

Figure 3-4 Annual sex- and age-specific incidence rates of slipped capital femoral epiphysis, Connecticut, by age at diagnosis.

Source: Kelsey (83).

instance, in Connecticut the ratio of males to females was found to be 2.7 to 1 (83), while in Southwestern United States it was 1.7 to 1 (86).

In males, the left hip is affected twice as often as the right, while the right and left hips of females are affected with approximately equal frequency (22,78,82,90). In both sexes, about 20 to 25 percent of slipped epiphysis cases have both hips affected (22,66,78,82,139).

The incidence of slipped epiphysis is greater in blacks than in whites. In Connecticut, estimates of annual incidence rates per 100,000 in those under age 25 were 7.8 for black males, 6.7 for black females, 4.7 for white males, and 1.6 for white females (83). Within the United States, slipped

PERCENTAGE WITH WEIGHTS AT OR ABOVE
95th PERCENTILE FOR THEIR AGE

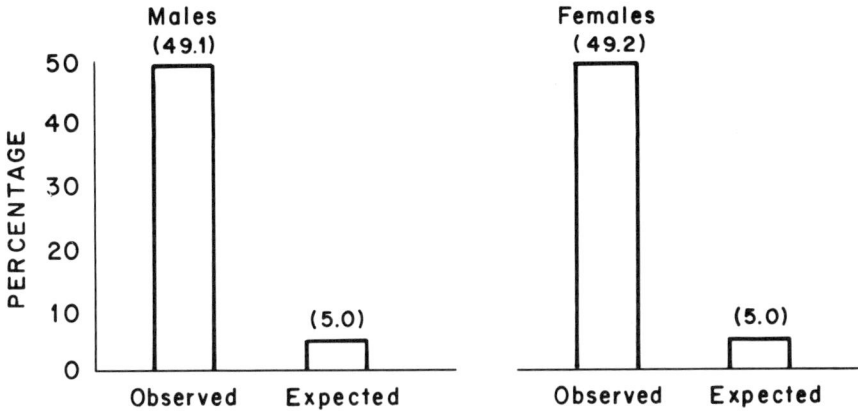

Figure 3-5 Percentage of cases of slipped femoral epiphysis with weights at or above the 95th percentile for their age.

Source: Kelsey et al. (85).

epiphysis is rarely diagnosed in the Southwestern and Rocky Mountain states, but is more frequently seen in the Midwestern, Southwestern, and North Central states (82). Urban-rural differences in incidence appear to be slight (83,86).

Several investigators have reported that symptoms begin more frequently in spring and summer than in autumn and winter (4,45,82,107), but this has not been found in all localities (86,139). The peak in spring and summer cannot be attributed to the seasonal distribution of related trauma or to the time of diagnosis of the slipped epiphysis (4,82).

A large proportion of slipped epiphysis patients are overweight (22,85,107,157). In Connecticut (85), 49 percent of both male and female patients with slipped epiphysis had weights at or above the 95th percentile for their age; 73 percent of males and 52 percent of females had weights at or above the 90th percentile for their height (Figure 3-5). There is also a tendency of slipped epiphysis patients to be tall for their age (22,45,85,139). However, little evidence exists (22,85,139) for the formerly held belief that tall thin children are particularly susceptible to slipped epiphysis.

Children with slipped epiphysis tend to have undergone slower-than-average skeletal maturation as indicated in X-rays of their hands

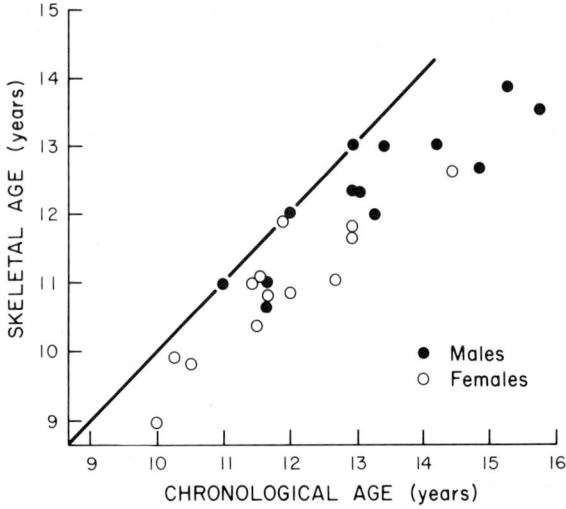

Figure 3-6 Skeletal age of cases of slipped capital femoral epiphysis according to chronological age.

Source: Morscher (107).

(107,120,139). Figure 3-6 shows that this trend is particularly marked among children of older chronological age.

Familial aggregation of cases has occasionally been reported (78,82,121), but it is not known whether this is primarily attributable to inherited characteristics or to environmental factors to which members of the same family are exposed.

Many of the risk factors for slipped epiphysis are associated with either a weakening of the epiphyseal plate or an increase in the shearing stress on the plate. A weakened epiphyseal plate, for instance, occurs during periods of rapid growth, such as during the adolescent growth spurt (107). Males have a greater and longer-lasting growth spurt than females and the male growth spurt is more likely to be characterized by periods of growth retardation in response to environmental stresses such as starvation or disease, followed by periods of rapid growth (1). Also, it has been reported (102,107,124,144) that growth of children is more rapid in spring and summer than in fall and winter; this might explain the excess of onset of symptoms in spring and summer.

In addition, certain hormones influence the strength of the epiphyseal plate. A variety of endocrinopathies are occasionally seen in patients with slipped epiphysis (115), but the effects of growth hormone and sex hormones on the epiphyseal plate have received the most consideration. Animal experiments indicate that a deficit of sex hormones relative to growth hormone brings about a widening of the epiphyseal plate and a reduction in the shearing force necessary to displace the epiphysis (63,107). Accordingly, slowly maturing children may be more likely to develop the disease because they are exposed for a longer period of time to high levels of growth hormone relative to sex hormones than fast maturers are. Tall children also have a longer-than-average exposure to growth hormone with relatively low levels of sex hormones. The occurrence of slipped epiphysis during treatment of children with growth hormone has been reported (48,122). The observation that estrogens protect against slipped epiphysis while androgens are protective only in larger doses after prolonged exposure (68,107) may be another reason for the higher incidence in males than females.

The shearing stress to which the epiphyseal plate is exposed is another important factor. The plate changes from a horizontal to an oblique plane during adolescence, so that it becomes more vulnerable to stress from superincumbent weight. Since overweight children have more superincumbent weight than lighter ones, the additional shearing stress in these children is probably one of the major reasons they have the disease more frequently. It is also possible that the left hip of males is for some reason subject to more shearing stress than the right and that the hips of blacks are in a position more vulnerable to stress than those of whites, but so far little evidence exists to support or refute these possibilities. Shearing stress from forward movement in such activities as walking or running may also be of some etiologic significance.

It was once believed that direct physical trauma to the hip was an important cause of slipped epiphysis (56,147), but it is now realized that in the majority of instances, trauma is at most only a minor contributing factor. When trauma does appear to precipitate the slipped epiphysis, the trauma is usually no greater than that experienced by all children in the course of their daily lives.

Finally, the combined effects of increased shearing stress and a weakened epiphyseal plate must be especially great. It has been suggested without any empirical evidence (84) that a child who has the unusual combination of being overweight and undergoing slow skeletal maturation would be especially vulnerable. Also, another reason for the male excess of cases may be that they generally develop slipped epiphysis at a later chronological age than females, so that they tend to weigh more at their time of maximum vulnerability.

Thus, most of the risk factors for slipped epiphysis, including the adolescent age group, the male sex, the states of being overweight, tall, and undergoing slow skeletal maturation, and the excess of symptoms in spring and summer, can be related to hormones or increased mechanical stress. The reasons for the higher incidence in blacks than whites and for the larger number of cases affecting the left hip than the right in males but not in females, however, are not known. Studies of asymmetry in the left and right hips of males and females would be of interest. Also, the hypothesis that being both overweight and a slow maturer makes one susceptible should be specifically tested.

SCHEUERMANN'S DISEASE

In Scheuermann's disease there is a kyphosis, or an increase in the posterior convex curvature, of the thoracic spine. In severe cases, this results in a hunchback appearance. Scheuermann's disease is often painless, although there may be minor backache. Three to five adjacent vertebrae in the middle and lower parts of the thoracic spine are generally affected, and the affected area is rigid. On examination, there is a "round-shouldered" appearance, a rounded prominence in the thoracic region, and compensatory cervical and lumbar lordosis. On X-ray, anterior wedging of one or more vertebra(e), irregular vertebral end plates, narrowing of the disc spaces, and a thoracic kyphosis may be seen (15,16). Kyphosis can result from congenital abnormalities, paralytic diseases, infectious diseases affecting the spine, hereditary diseases, spinal surgery, and certain metabolic diseases such as osteoporosis. However, the present discussion is limited to idiopathic adolescent kyphosis, known as Scheuermann's disease.

The thoracic spine normally has a certain degree of posterior convex curvature. The decision as to when the extent of this curvature is abnormal is somewhat subjective. Scheuermann (134) defined pathologic kyphosis as curvature greater than 35° in the thoracic spine, whereas Bradford et al. (18) set the limit of normal curvature at 40°. Prevalence rates are accordingly influenced considerably by the definition of the disease.

Estimates of the prevalence of Scheuermann's disease have ranged from 4 to 8 percent; these estimates have used various diagnostic criteria and are all based on findings in men entering or enlisting into the armed services (36,52,148). Among cases seeking treatment, some investigators have found more males than females (26,69), while others have reported a female preponderance (15,70,110). The most common ages at onset are between 10 and 14 years of age (15,70), with the peak incidence in girls occurring about two to three years earlier than in boys (70,110).

Although tall and thin individuals are reported to have a greater risk than those who are short and stocky (70), no data have been published to support this contention. Familial aggregation of Scheuermann's disease has generally not been found, although occasionally isolated families with many affected members have been described (13,61).

The causes of Scheuermann's disease are not known. Various theories have been put forth, but none has gained general acceptance. The disorder was first described as a disease caused by avascular necrosis of the "vertebral epiphyses" that would lead to growth inhibition and a subsequent kyphotic curve (134). However, it is now known that the "epiphyseal ring" is not a true epiphysis and does not take an active part in longitudinal growth of the vertebral body. Instead, some disruption of the actual epiphyseal growth plates may cause the kyphotic curve (11,12).

Schmorl and Junghanns (135) and others (92,123) have proposed that herniation of disc material through weakened spots in the cartilaginous growth plates causes disruption of the growth plate. The resulting loss of disc height would increase the flexion of the thoracic region of the spine; this would then put more pressure on the anterior portion of the vertebral body (91). The result would be wedging of vertebrae and a fixed kyphotic curve (135). Herniation of disc material into the growth plates of individuals with kyphotic curves has been reported (8,69,135), but such herniations (called Schmorl's nodes) may also be found in areas of the spine not included in the kyphotic curve of affected individuals as well as in the spines of individuals without Scheuermann's disease (15). To take these observations into account, Hilton et al. (69) and Stoddard and Osborn (143) have suggested that it is only the severe herniations that result in Scheuermann's disease, and Resnick and Niwayama (123) postulated that there is a genetic predisposition to weakened cartilaginous end plates. However, these suggestions have not been substantiated by data.

Biomechanical aspects of the spine have also received attention. White and colleagues (150) have pointed out that impairment of either the compression-resisting anterior elements or the tension-resisting posterior elements of the spine may produce a kyphotic curve. Because of the natural kyphotic curve in the thoracic region and because the tension-resisting capsules of the facet joints are less well developed in the thoracic spine than in other regions, the likelihood of occurrence of Scheuermann's disease is increased if the compression-resisting anterior elements are impaired. It has also been suggested that physical stress on the spine from manual labor or from trauma contributes to the development of the disease (134,148), and that short hamstring muscles make a child more susceptible to flexion injuries (92). However, studies are needed to evaluate these hypotheses.

The role of diet in the etiology of Scheuermann's disease has been considered. Fluorides in drinking water do not appear to be related to the prevalence of the disease (87,88), and normal levels of serum calcium, phosphorus, vitamin A, and vitamin C have been reported in patients with Scheuermann's disease (110). However, Bradford et al. (17) found that family members of twelve cases of Scheuermann's disease reported less intake of foods high in calcium than families of twenty adolescents who had died of acute trauma, but it is not known whether the cases and controls were comparable in other relevant respects. These investigators suggested that Scheuermann's disease is a form of juvenile osteoporosis. Experiments in rats suggested that vitamin E deficiency increases the likelihood of occurrence of kyphoscoliosis (100), but this has apparently not been evaluated in humans. Thus, evidence that diet plays a role in the etiology of Scheuermann's disease is not strong, but the possibility cannot be excluded at this time.

Both basic descriptive data and studies to test specific hypotheses are needed. Individuals with and without Scheuermann's disease should be compared according to such basic demographic variables as ethnicity and social class, according to height and weight as determined from actual measurements, and according to skeletal maturation status and age at menarche. Hypotheses concerning the possible etiologic role of severe Schmorl's nodes, of biomechanical factors, and of physical activity need to be evaluated by laboratory and epidemiologic studies. Obtaining data on dietary factors in affected and unaffected individuals will be difficult, and much larger numbers of subjects are needed if any actual differences are to be detected.

SCOLIOSIS

This is an abnormal lateral curvature of the spine (see Figure 3-7). The main curve is called the primary curve, while the secondary curves, which may occur both above and below the primary curve, develop to compensate for the imbalance caused by the primary curve. Scoliosis may be categorized into three main types (Table 3-2). Nonstructural scoliosis has

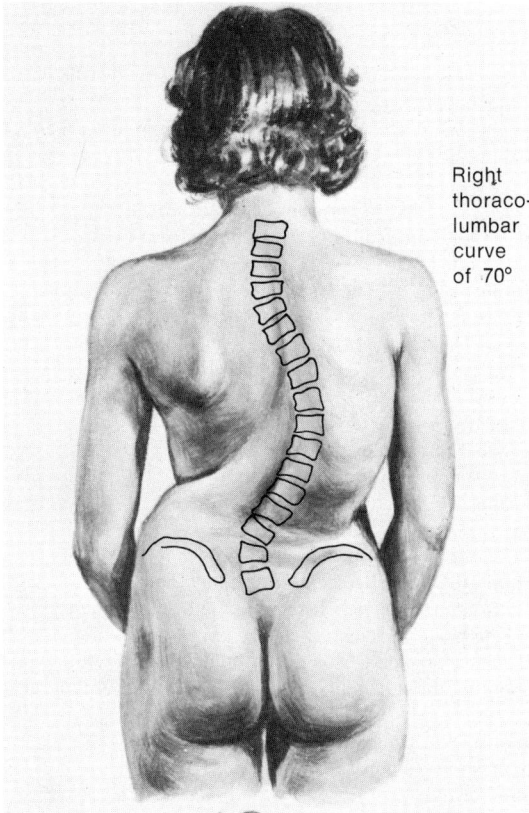

Figure 3-7 Scoliosis: Right thoracolumbar curve of 70°.

Source: Keim (81). © Copyright 1978 CIBA Pharmaceutical Company, Division of CIBA-GEIGY Corporation. Reprinted with permission from *Clinical Symposia,* illustrated by Frank Netter, M.D. All rights reserved.

no "fixed" curve, and normal alignment would result if a patient were to hang by his or her hands. This type of scoliosis may occur, for instance, because the spine is held tilted or because of leg length discrepancy. Transient structural scoliosis occurs in response to some temporary condition such as a herniated disc. Structural scoliosis is present at all times when it occurs and would remain even if a person were to hang by his or her hands. Table 3-2 indicates that structural scoliosis can be further subclassified according to different causes. Idiopathic scoliosis is by far the largest category of structural scoliosis, and it is the focus of this discussion.

Idiopathic scoliosis may develop any time during the years of growth

Table 3-2   Classification of Scoliosis

I. Nonstructural Scoliosis

A. Postural Scoliosis. Usually noted in later years of first decade. Curves are always slight and disappear on lying down
B. Compensatory Scoliosis. Usually a result of leg length discrepancy. Pelvis dips down on the short side

II. Transient Structural Scoliosis

A. Sciatic Scoliosis. Not true scoliosis; an irritative form caused by pressure on nerve roots from a herniated disc
B. Hysterical Scoliosis. Rare, usually requires psychiatric treatment
C. Inflammatory Scoliosis. Seen with perinephric abscess or similar infection

III. Structural Scoliosis

A. Idiopathic Scoliosis. About 70% of all cases of scoliosis. Classified by age of onset
   1. Infantile—before 3 years of age
   2. Juvenile—age 3 to onset of puberty, usually age 10
   3. Adolescent—from age 10 until maturity
B. Congenital Scoliosis
   1. Vertebral
     a. Open—with posterior spinal defect
       i. with neurologic deficit (e.g., myelomeningocele)
       ii. without neurologic deficit (e.g., spina bifida occulta)
     b. Closed—no posterior element defect
       i. with neurologic deficit (e.g., diastematomyelia with spina bifida)
       ii. without neurologic deficit (e.g., hemivertebra, unilateral unsegmented bar)
   2. Extravertebral (e.g., congenital rib fusions)
C. Neuromuscular Scoliosis
   1. Neuropathic forms
     a. Lower motor neuron disease (e.g., poliomyelitis)
     b. Upper motor neuron disease (e.g., cerebral palsy)
     c. Others (e.g., syringomyelia)
   2. Myopathic forms
     a. Progressive (e.g., muscular dystrophy)
     b. Static (e.g., amyotonia congenita)
   3. Others (e.g., Friedreich's ataxia, unilateral amelia)
D. Neurofibromatosis (von Recklinghausen's disease)
E. Mesenchymal Disorders
   1. Congenital (e.g., Marfan's syndrome, Morquio's disease, amyoplasia congenita, various types of dwarfism)
   2. Acquired (e.g., rheumatoid arthritis, Still's disease)
   3. Others (e.g., Scheuermann's disease, osteogenesis imperfecta)
F. Trauma
   1. Vertebral (e.g., fracture, irradiation, surgery)
   2. Extravertebral (e.g., burns, thoracic surgery)

Source: Keim (81).

from infancy through adolescence, and may be further subdivided according to the age of onset and by the location of the curve within the spine (thoracic, thoracolumbar, double thoracic, thoracic, cervicothoracic, and double primary curves affecting the thoracic and lumbar spines). Infantile scoliosis generally affects children less than 4 years of age; juvenile scoliosis by definition occurs after age 3 but before the onset of puberty, and adolescent scoliosis is seen most frequently in the age range 10 to 18 years (74,158).

Estimates of the prevalence of scoliosis are influenced by (1) the age group studied, (2) the degree of curvature considered pathologic, (3) whether the diagnosis is made by X-ray or physical examination, and (4) the part of the spine that is X-rayed, if X-rays are taken. Furthermore, the definition of scoliosis used may depend on whether the objective is to determine prevalence, to identify cases in need of treatment, or to detect all measurable curves. Consequently, reports of prevalence rates in the United States range from 1 per 1000 to 14 per 100 (38,80,97,137), the lower rates based on cases referred to orthopedists for treatment and the higher on children with curves of 5° or more in the general population. Typical prevalence rates are those based on an evaluation of curves from chest X-rays of 50,000 people of age 14 years or older in Delaware. The prevalence of curves of 10° to 19° was 1.4 percent; of curves of 20° to 29°, 0.3 percent; and of curves 30° or greater, 0.2 percent (137). Of all these curves, 92 percent were idiopathic. All studies have found that slight curves are considerably more common than larger curves. Kane (79) in fact found that prevalence rates by degree of curvature follow a log-normal distribution.

Infantile idiopathic scoliosis may be considered a mild form of the disorder, since regression of the curve occurs spontaneously in about 90 percent of cases (75,81). It is seen much more commonly in Great Britain than in the United States. Data on its relative frequency in the two areas are available from a collaborative survey undertaken in Boston, Massachusetts (126), and Edinburgh, Scotland (160), in which one-third of idiopathic scoliosis patients in Edinburgh but only 0.5 percent in Boston were infantile onset. Scoliosis with infantile onset is more common in males than females, and 90 percent of the curves are to the left (75,81,160). Theories as to causes of infantile scoliosis include vitamin D deficiency, poor nutrition, lack of sunlight (127), and asymmetric maturation of the neuromuscular components of the spine (23), but none of these is well established.

Juvenile-onset scoliosis is less common than infantile-onset or adoles-

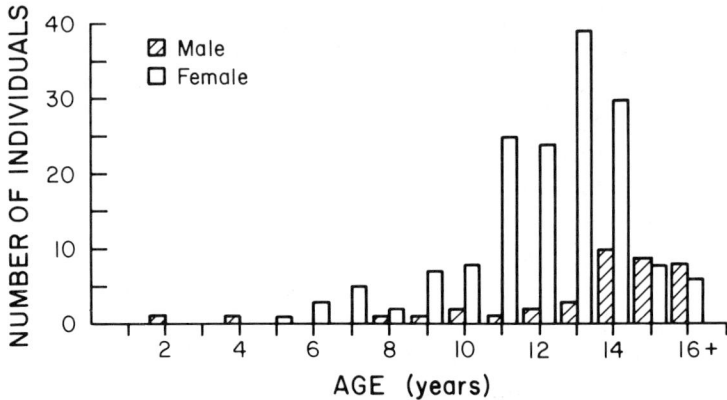

Figure 3-8 Age at onset, by history, of idiopathic scoliosis, 208 patients.

Source: Riseborough and Wynne-Davies (126).

cent-onset scoliosis, but in general the curves do not disappear spontaneously. Little is known of its epidemiology.

Adolescent idiopathic scoliosis is the most common cause of spine
deformity seen in North American children (158). Severity varies considerably, and it is difficult at present to predict which curves will progress
(158). Treatment usually involves some combination of bedrest, exercise,
traction, and a plaster cast or brace, although surgery may be necessary
in some cases. Individuals who are left with significant curvature frequently develop spinal osteoarthrosis as adults, and if untreated, lung and
heart complications are likely (14,108).

Figure 3-8 shows that females are most frequently affected around the
ages of 11 to 14 years and males at about 14 to 16 years (126). Although
at surgery the ratio of female to male cases is as high as 5 to 1 (158), the
overall female excess is attributable to the greater number of females with
severe curves; the milder curves of 5° to 15° are found with almost equal
frequency in males and females (9,20,129,138,140). In one study, the
female to male ratio was 1.0 to 1 for curves of 6° to 10°, 1.4 to 1 for
curves of 11° to 20°, and 5.4 to 1 for curves of 20° or more (129). About
90 percent of adolescent-onset curves are to the right (75,81,160).

Little is known of the prevalence of adolescent scoliosis according to
race. Shands and Eisberg (137) found no overall difference in prevalence
rates between blacks and whites among Delaware residents of age 14
years and over, but found that blacks tended to have a greater proportion
of moderate and severe curves and whites of slight curves. Among school-

children in Johannesburg, South Africa, however, the prevalence of scoliosis of 10° or more as determined by X-ray was found to be higher in whites than blacks (136).

Familial aggregation of idiopathic adolescent scoliosis has long been noted. Disagreement exists as to the extent to which this results from genetic or environmental factors, and if genetic, the specific mode of inheritance. In a few families with many affected members, it is felt that some genetic metabolic error must be involved (54,128). In most families, however, the degree of familial aggregation is less marked. In these families the prevalence is greatest in first-degree relatives of cases, followed by second-degree relatives, with the prevalence in third-degree relatives similar to or slightly higher than that found in the general population (50,126,160). If both parents have idiopathic scoliosis, the likelihood that their offspring will develop a curve needing treatment is 50 times greater than that in the general population (99). Several investigators have found that relatives of female scoliosis patients were more often affected by scoliosis than relatives of male patients (35,37,126,160), but the reasons for this are not known.

Available evidence suggests that polygenic inheritance with strong influence from environmental factors is the correct genetic model in most cases. The higher than expected prevalence in first and to a certain extent second degree relatives, the greater variance in the degree of curvature among dizygotic than among monozygotic twin pairs (37), and the higher concordance among monozygotic twins than among dizygotic pairs tend to support a polygenic model (33).

Much attention has been focused on the role of skeletal growth and maturation in the etiology of adolescent idiopathic scoliosis, since curves progress very rapidly around the time of adolescent growth spurt, and since females are on the average affected about two years earlier than males. Both boys and girls with scoliosis are taller but not heavier than other individuals of the same age at the beginning of adolescence; however, at the end of adolescence, the girls are no longer taller than average (Figure 3-9), although there is still some difference in the boys (Figure 3-10) (113,152,153,155,156). It is not clear whether the tendency of scoliosis cases to be taller is due to greater length of the spine or to greater total height (98,154). Scoliotic females have been observed to have a faster rate of growth around ages 8 and 9 years than others of their age, but by 11 years their rate of growth is similar to that of others of their age (152,155). The same trend is seen in males at a slightly later age, but to a lesser degree. Age at menarche of female cases has been found to be

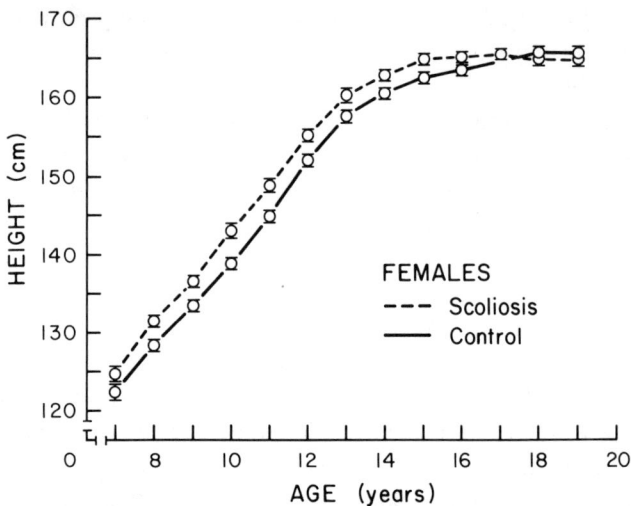

Figure 3-9   Mean heights of girls with and without scoliosis.
Source: Willner (152).

Figure 3-10   Mean heights of boys with and without scoliosis.
Source: Willner (152).

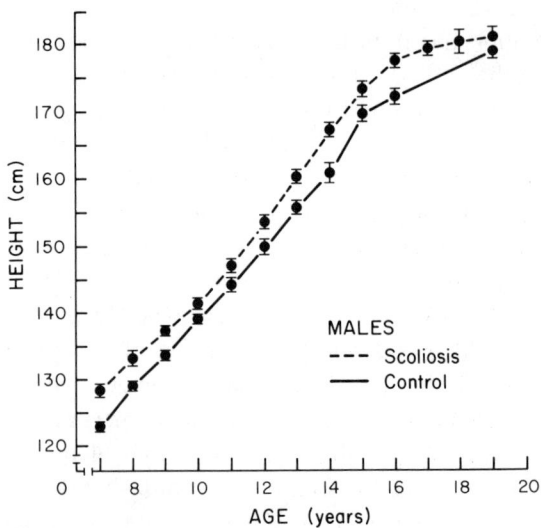

similar to that of controls, again suggesting that their rate of maturation slows after its initial fast start (29,98,153). When skeletal maturation is estimated by X-ray, scoliotic girls are more mature than the average girl in early adolescence, but are less skeletally mature by about age 15 years (98,113). Similar studies of males have not been undertaken. Thus, the data consistently indicate that those who develop scoliosis mature more rapidly than others in early adolescence, but that their rate of maturation slows subsequently.

Interest in the relationship of patterns of growth to scoliosis has led several investigators to study levels of hormones that influence growth, such as growth hormones and estrogens. However, to date studies have not shown much difference in hormone levels between individuals with scoliosis and others of their age and sex (104,156).

It has also been suggested that idiopathic scoliosis may result from mechanical stress on a functional curve. In one study, a shorter left than right leg was found in 80 percent of young children; this was hypothesized to result in left lumbar and right thoracic curves, the thoracic curve eventually becoming structural (109). It is known that most individuals in the general population have a slight right thoracic curve (44,149). White and Panjabi (149) have postulated that some imbalance in this slight curvature might result in asymmetrical loading and muscle imbalance, with the subsequent development of a structural curve in some individuals.

Defects in the spinal musculature have been considered in the etiology of scoliosis. For instance, increased muscle activity has been found on the convex side of the scoliotic curve at the apex (3,27,60,67,95,125,145,164), an asymmetry that is found in those with idiopathic or paralytic scoliosis, but not in postural or congenital scoliosis (67,125). It has also been reported that the greater the degree of curvature, the greater the electrical activity on the convex side and that the asymmetrical activity is apparent in progressing but not in nonprogressing curves (164). Evidence is inconclusive as to whether there are differences in the type of muscle fiber in the spinal musculature that could contribute to the development of scoliosis (49,141,142). These studies in humans do not permit one to know whether the change in muscle activity preceded or resulted from the scoliosis, but evidence from experiments in animals does indicate that scoliosis can be induced by altering spinal musculature (93,116).

Equilibrium dysfunction has been suggested to be associated with adolescent idiopathic scoliosis (76,109,130–132,162,163). Sahlstrand et al. (132), for instance, performed tests on scoliotic patients which led them to believe that persons with scoliosis may have a dysfunction either in the labyrinth system of the ear or in the brain stem where the postural control mechanisms are located. Again, it is impossible to know whether the equilibrium dysfunctions are causes or effects of the disease.

Finally, the role of metabolic factors has been considered. Disorders of collagen have been suggested to be related to scoliosis (6,10,25,53,112), but there is evidence that some of these changes may be secondary to the scoliosis (25,117). Also, it is not clear why these disorders of collagen would result only in a spinal defect and not in a more generalized skeletal disorder.

In summary, adolescent idiopathic scoliosis occurs at the time of the adolescent growth spurt, and affects females more often than males, at least in its severe form. Also, the prevalence is highest in those who are skeletally more mature at the onset but not at the end of puberty. Similarly, individuals with scoliosis tend to be taller and leaner than others of their age at the beginning but not at the end of adolescence, especially among females. There seems to be some genetic predisposition to scoliosis. The etiologic roles of biomechanical, muscular, and metabolic factors and of equilibrium disorders have yet to be firmly elucidated.

REFERENCES

1. Acheson, R. M. 1966. "Maturation of the skeleton." In *Human Development*. F. Falkner, ed. Philadelphia: Saunders.
2. Al-Aswad, B. I., Weinger, B. I., and Schneider, A. B. 1978. "Slipped capital femoral epiphysis in a 35 year old man." *Clin. Orthop.* 134:131–134.
3. Alexander, M. A., and Season, E. H. 1978. "Idiopathic scoliosis: An electromyographic study." *Arch. Phys. and Rehab.* 59:314–315.
4. Andrèn, L., and Borgshom, K. 1958. "Seasonal variation of epiphysiolysis of the hip and possibility of a causal factor." *Acta Orthop. Scand.* 28:22–26.
5. Aston, J. N. 1967. *A Short Textbook of Orthopaedics and Traumatology.* Philadelphia: Lippincott.
6. Balaba, T. Y. 1972. "Some biochemical aspects of scoliosis and their pathogenetic significance." *Reconstr. Surg. Traumat.* 13:191–209.
7. Barker, D. J. P., Dixon, E., and Taylor, J. F. 1978. "Perthes' disease of the hip in three regions of England." *J. Bone Jt. Surg. (Brit.)* 60:478–480.
8. Batts, M., Jr. 1939. "Rupture of the nucleus pulposus. An anatomical study." *J. Bone Jt. Surg.* 21:121–126.
9. Bellyei,A., Cziezel, A., Barta, O., Magda, T., and Molnar, L. 1977. "Prevalence of adolescent idiopathic scoliosis in Hungary." *Acta Orthop. Scand.* 48:177–180.
10. Benson, P. F. 1972. "Hydroxyproline excretion in idiopathic, congenital and paralytic scoliosis (letter)." *Arch. Dis. Child.* 47:476.
11. Bick, E. M., and Copel, J. W. 1950. "Longitudinal growth of the human vertebra. A contribution to human osteogeny." *J. Bone Jt. Surg. (Amer.)* 32:803–814.

12. ———, and Copel, J. W. 1951. "The ring apophysis of the human vertebra." *J. Bone Jt. Surg. (Amer.)* 33:783–787.
13. Bjersand, A. J. 1980. "Juvenile kyphosis in identical twins." *Amer. J. Roent.* 134:598–599.
14. Bjure, J., Grimby, G., Kasalicky, J., Lindh, M., and Nachemson, A. 1970. "Respiratory impairment and airway closure in patients with untreated idiopathic scoliosis." *Thorax* 25:451–456.
15. Bradford, D. S. 1977. "Juvenile kyphosis." *Clin. Orthop.* 128:45–55.
16. ———. 1975. "Scheuermann's juvenile kyphosis. A histologic study." *Clin. Orthop.* 110:45–53.
17. ———, Brown, D. M., Moe, J. H., and Winter, R. B. 1976. "Scheuermann's kyphosis. A form of osteoporosis?" *Clin. Orthop.* 118:10–15.
18. ———, Brown, D. M., Montalvo, F. J., and Winter, B. B. 1974. "Scheuermann's kyphosis and round back deformity." *J. Bone Jt. Surg. (Amer.)* 56:740–758.
19. Breck, L. W. 1971. *An Atlas of the Osteochondroses.* Springfield, Ill.: Charles C Thomas.
20. Brooks, H. L., Azen, S. D., Gerberg, E., Brooks, R., and Chan, L. 1975. "Scoliosis: A prospective epidemiological study." *J. Bone Jt. Surg. (Amer.)* 57:968–972.
21. Bruns, D. 1960. "Hüftkopfepiphysenlösung bei einem 22-jährigen mann mit hormonell gestörtem wachstum." *Zeit Orthop.* 92:453–457.
22. Burrows, H. J. 1957. "Slipped upper femoral epiphysis." *J. Bone Jt. Surg. (Brit.)* 39:641–658.
23. Burwell, R. G. 1971. "The relationship between scoliosis and growth." In *Scoliosis and Growth.* P. A. Zorab, ed. London: Churchill and Livingstone, pp. 131–150.
24. ———, Dangerfield, P. H., Hall, D. J., Vernon, C. L., and Harrison, M. H. M. 1978. "Perthes' Disease. An anthropometric study revealing impaired and disproportionate growth." *J. Bone Jt. Surg. (Brit.)* 60:461–477.
25. Bushell, G. R., Ghosh, P., Taylor, T. K. F., and Sutherland, J. M. 1979. "The collagen of the intervertebral disc in adolescent idiopathic scoliosis." *J. Bone Jt. Surg. (Brit.)* 61:501–508.
26. Butler, R. W. 1955. "The nature and significance of vertebral osteochondritis." *Proc. Roy. Soc. Med.* 48:895–902.
27. Butterworth, T. R., and James, C. 1969. "Electromyographic studies in idiopathic scoliosis." *Southern Med. J.* 62:1008–1010.
28. Caffey, J. 1968. "The early roentgenographic changes in essential coxa plana: Their significance in pathogenesis." *Amer. J. of Roentgenology* 103:620–634.
29. Calvo, I. J. 1957. "Observations on the growth of the female adolescent spine and its relation to scoliosis." *Clin. Orthop.* 10:40–47.
30. Cameron, J. M., and Izatt, M. M. 1960. "Legg-Calvé-Perthes disease." *Scot. Med. J.* 5:148–154.
31. Catterall, A., Lloyd-Roberts, G. C., and Wynne-Davies, R. 1971. "Association of Perthes' disease with congenital anomalies of genitourinary tract and inguinal region." *Lancet* 1:996–997.
32. Cavanaugh, L. A., Shelton, E. K., and Sutherland, R. 1936. "Metabolic studies in osteochondritis of the capital femoral epiphysis." *J. Bone Jt. Surg.* 18:957–968.
33. Cowell, H. R., Hall, J. N., and MacEwen, G. D. 1972. "Genetic aspects of idiopathic scoliosis." *Clin. Orthop.* 86:121–131.
34. Cozen, L. 1962. "Theoretical considerations on the etiology of Legg-Calvé-Perthes disease and slipped femoral capital epiphysis." *Arch. Pediat.* 79:115–118.

35. Czeizel, A., Bellyei, Á., Barta, O., Magda, T., and Molnar, L. 1978. "Genetics of adolescent idiopathic scoliosis." *J. Med. Genet.* 15:424–427.

36. Dameron, T. B., and Gulledge, W. H. 1953. "Adolescent kyphosis." *U.S. Armed Forces Med. J.* 4:871–875.

37. DeGeorge, F. V., and Fisher, R. L. 1967. "Idiopathic scoliosis: Genetic and environmental aspects." *J. Med. Genet.* 4:251–257.

38. Drennan, J. C., Campbell, J. B., and Ridge, H. 1977. "Denver: A metropolitan public school scoliosis survey." *Pediatrics* 60:193–196.

39. Ebong, W. W. 1977. "Legg-Calvé-Perthes disease in Nigerians." *Int. Surg.* 62(4):217–218.

40. Edgren, W. 1965. "Coxa plana: A clinical and radiological investigation with particular reference to the importance of the metaphyseal changes for the final shape of the proximal part of the femur." *Acta Orthop. Scand. Suppl.* 84:1–129.

41. Ehrenborg, G. 1962. "The Osgood-Schlatter lesion. A clinical and experimental study." *Acta Chir. Scand. Suppl.* 288.

42. ———, Engfeldt, B., and Olsson, S. E. 1961. "On the aetiology of the Osgood-Schlatter lesion. An experimental study in dogs." *Acta Chir. Scand.* 122:445–457.

43. ———, and Lagergren, C. 1961. "The normal arterial pattern of tuberositas tibiae in adolescents and in growing dogs." *Acta Chir. Scand.* 121:500–510.

44. Farkas, A. 1941. "Physiological scoliosis." *J. Bone Jt. Surg.* 23:607–627.

45. Ferguson, A. B., and Howorth, B. 1931. "Slipping of the upper femoral epiphysis." *J. Amer. Med. Ass.* 97:1–867.

46. ———, and Howorth, M. B. 1934. "Coxa plana and related conditions of the hip." *J. Bone Jt. Surg.* 16:781–803.

47. Ferguson, A. B., Jr. 1975. *Orthopaedic Surgery in Infancy and Childhood.* Baltimore: Williams and Wilkins.

48. Fidler, M. W., and Brook, C. G. B. 1974. "Slipped upper femoral epiphysis following treatment with human growth hormone." *J. Bone Jt. Surg. (Amer.)* 56:1719–1722.

49. ———and Jowett, R. L. 1976. "Muscle imbalance in the aetiology of scoliosis." *J. Bone Jt. Surg. (Brit.)* 58:200–201.

50. Filho, N. A., and Thompson, M. W. 1971. "Genetic studies in scoliosis." (News Notes) *J. Bone Jt. Surg. (Amer.)* 53:199.

51. Fisher, R. 1972. "An epidemiological study of Legg-Calvé-Perthes disease." *J. Bone Jt. Surg. (Amer.)* 54:769–778.

52. Fletcher, G. H. 1947. "Anterior vertebral wedging—Frequency and significance." *Am. J. Roent.* 57:232–238.

53. Francis, M. J., Smith, R., and Sanderson, M. C. 1977. "Collagen abnormalities in idiopathic adolescent scoliosis." *Calcif. Tissue Res.* (Suppl.) 22:381–384.

54. Garland, H. G. 1934. "Hereditary scoliosis." *Brit. Med. J.* 1:328.

55. Garn, S. M., Rohmann, C. G., and Silverman, F. N. 1967. "Radiographic standards for postnatal ossification and tooth calcification." *Med. Rad. and Photo.* 43:45–66.

56. Ghormley, R. K., and Fairchild, R. D. 1940. "The diagnosis and treatment of slipped epiphysis." *J. Amer. Med. Ass.* 114:229–235.

57. Goff, C. W. 1954. *Legg-Calvé-Perthes Syndrome and Related Osteochondrosis of Youth.* Springfield, Ill.: Charles C Thomas.

58. Golding, J. S. R., MacIves, J. E., and Wont, L. N. 1959. "The bone changes in sickle-cell anemia and its genetic variants." *J. Bone Jt. Surg. (Brit.)* 41:711–718.

59. Gray, J. M., Lowry, R. B., and Renwick, D. H. G. 1972. "Incidence and genetics of Legg-Perthes disease (osteochondritis deformans) in British Columbia: Evidence of polygenic determination." *J. Med. Genet.* 9:197–202.

60. Gruca, A. 1958. "The pathogenesis and treatment of idiopathic scoliosis. A preliminary report." *J. Bone Jt. Surg. (Amer.)* 40:570–584.

61. Halal, F., Gledhill, R. B., and Fraser, C. 1978. "Dominant inheritance of Scheuermann's juvenile kyphosis." *Amer. J. Dis. Child* 132:1105–1107.

62. Harper, P., Brotherton, B. J., and Cochlin, D. 1976. "Genetic risks in Perthes' disease." *Clinical Genetics* 10:178–182.

63. Harris, W. R. 1950. "The endocrine basis for slipping of the upper femoral epiphysis: An experimental study." *J. Bone Jt. Surg. (Brit.)* 32:5–11.

64. ———, and Hobson, K. W. 1956. "Histological changes in experimentally displaced upper femoral epiphysis in rabbits." *J. Bone Jt. Surg. (Brit.)* 38:914–921.

65. Harrison, M. H. M., Turner, M. H., and Jacobs, P. 1976. "Skeletal immaturity in Perthes disease." *J. Bone Jt. Surg. (Brit.)* 58:37–40.

66. Henrikson, B. 1969. "The incidence of slipped capital femoral epiphysis." *Acta Orthop. Scand.* 40:365–372.

67. Henssge, J. 1968. "Are signs of denervation of the muscles of the spine primary or secondary findings in cases of scoliosis?" *J. Bone Jt. Surg. (Brit.)* 50:882.

68. Hillman, J. W., Hunter, W. A., Jr., and Barrow, J. A. 1957. "Experimental epiphysiolysis in rats." *Surgical Forum* 8:566–571.

69. Hilton, R. C., Ball, J., and Bean, R. T. 1976. "Vertebral end-plate lesions (Schmorl's nodes) in the dorsolumbar spine." *Ann. Rheum. Dis.* 35:127–132.

70. Hodgen, J. T., and Frantz, C. H. 1941. "Juvenile kyphosis." *Surg. Gynecol. Obstet.* 72:798–806.

71. Hughes, E. S. R. 1948. "Osgood-Schlatter's disease." *Surg., Gynec. and Obstet.* 86:323–328.

72. Inoue, A., Freeman, M. A. R., Vernon-Roberts, and Mizuno, S. 1976. "The pathogenesis of Perthes' disease." *J. Bone Jt. Surg. (Brit.)* 58:453–461.

73. Jacobs, B. W. 1971. "Synovitis of the hip in children and its significance." *Pediatrics* 47:558–566.

74. James, J. I. P. 1954. "Idiopathic scoliosis: The prognosis, diagnosis, and operative indications related to curve patterns and the age at onset." *J. Bone Jt. Surg. (Brit.)* 36:36–49.

75. ———. 1970. "The etiology of scoliosis." *J. Bone Jt. Surg. (Brit.)* 52:410–419.

76. Jensen, G. M., and Wilson, K. B. 1979. "Horizontal postrotatory nystagmus response in female subjects with adolescent idiopathic scoliosis." *Phys. Ther.* 59:1226–1233.

77. Jensen, O. M., and Lauritzen, J. 1976. "Legg-Calvé Perthes disease. Morphological studies in two cases examined at necropsy." *J. Bone Jt. Surg. (Brit.)* 58:332–338.

78. Jerre, T. 1960. "A study in slipped upper femoral epiphysis." *Acta Orthop. Scand. Suppl.* 6:1–157.

79. Kane, W. J. 1977. "Scoliosis prevalence: A call for a statement of terms." *Clin. Orthop.* 126:43–46.

80. ———, and Moe, J. H. 1970. "A scoliosis-prevalence survey in Minnesota." *Clin. Orthop.* 69:216–218.

81. Keim, H. A. 1972. "Scoliosis." *CIBA Clinical Symposia.* 30:2–30.

82. Kelsey, J. L. 1969. "An epidemiological study of slipped capital femoral epiphysis." Thesis, Ph.D., Epidemiology and Public Health, Yale University.

83. ———. 1971. "Incidence and distribution of slipped capital femoral epiphysis in Connecticut." *J. Chronic Dis.* 23:567–578.

84. ———. 1973. "Epidemiology of slipped capital femoral epiphysis: A review of the literature." *Pediatrics* 1:1042–1050.

85. ———, Acheson, R. M., and Keggi, K. J. 1972. "The body builds of patients with slipped capital femoral epiphysis." *Amer. J. Dis. Child.* 124:276–281.
86. ———, Keggi, K. J., and Southwick, W. O. 1970. "The incidence and distribution of slipped capital femoral epiphysis in Connecticut and Southwestern United States." *J. Bone Jt. Surg. (Amer.)* 52:1203–1216.
87. Kemp, F. H., and Wilson, D. C. 1947. "Some factors in the aetiology of osteochondritis of the spine. A report on two families." *Brit. J. Radiol.* 20:410–417.
88. ———, Wilson, D. C., and Emrys-Rolaris, E. 1948. "Social and nutritional factors in adolescent osteochondritis of the spine." *Brit. J. Soc. Med.* 2:66–70.
89. Kemp. H. B. S. 1973. "Perthes' disease: An experimental and clinical study." *Ann. Roy. Coll. Surg. Engl.* 52:18–35.
90. Klein, A., Joplin, R. J., Reidy, J. A., and Hanelin, J. 1953. "Management of the contralateral hip in slipped capital femoral epiphysis." *J. Bone Jt. Surg. (Amer.)* 35:81–87.
91. Knutsson, F. 1948. "Observations on the growth of the vertebral body in Scheuermann's disease." *Acta Radiol.* 30:97–104.
92. Lambrinudi, C. 1934. "Adolescent and senile kyphosis." *Brit. Med. J.* 2:800–804.
93. Langenskiöld, A. 1971. "Growth disturbances in muscle: A possible factor in the pathogenesis of scoliosis." In *Scoliosis and Growth.* P. A. Zorab, ed. London: Churchill and Livingstone, pp. 85–90.
94. Lauritzen, J. 1975. "Legg-Calvé-Perthes disease: A comparative study." *Acta Ortho. Scand. Suppl.* 159.
95. LeFebvre, J., Triboulet-Chassevant, A., and Missirliu, M. F. 1962. "Electromyographic data in idiopathic scoliosis." *Arch. Phys. Med.* 42:710–711.
96. Ljunggien,G. 1967. "Legg-Calvé-Perthes disease in the dog." *Acta Orthop. Scand. Suppl.* 95.
97. Lonstein, J. E. 1977. "Screening for spinal deformities in Minnesota schools." *Clin. Orthop.* 126:33–42.
98. Low, W. D., Mok, C. K., Leong, J. C. Y., Yau, B. C., and Lisowski, F. P. 1978. "The development of southern Chinese girls with adolescent idiopathic scoliosis." *Spine* 3:152–156.
99. MacEwen, D., and Cowell, H. R. 1970. "Familial incidence of idiopathic scoliosis and its implications in patient treatment." *J. Bone Jt. Surg. (Amer.)* 52:405.
100. Machlin, L. J., Filipski, R., Nelson, J., Horn, L. R., and Brin, M. 1977. "Effects of a prolonged vitamin E deficiency in the rat." *J. Nutr.* 107:1200–1208.
101. Mau, H., and Schmitt, H. W. 1960. "Der konstitutionell-dysostotische Perthes und die skelettreifungshemmungen beim eigentlichen Perthes." *Zeitschrift fur Orthopaedie* 93:515–530.
102. McKee, J. P., and Eichorn, D. H. 1953. "Seasonal variations of physiological functions during adolescence." *Child Development* 24:225–234.
103. McKibbin, B., and Ralis, Z. 1974. "Pathological changes in a case of Perthes disease." *J. Bone Jt. Surg. (Brit.)* 56:438–447.
104. Misol, S., Ponseti, I. V., Samaan, N., and Bradbury, J. T. 1971. "Growth hormone blood levels in patients with idiopathic scoliosis." *Clin. Orthop.* 81:122–125.
105. Molloy, M. K., and MacMahon, B. 1966. "Incidence of Legg-Calvé-Perthes disease." *New Engl. J. Med.* 275:988–990.
106. ———, and MacMahon, B. 1967. "Birth weight and Legg-Calvé-Perthes disease." *J. Bone Jt. Surg. (Brit.)* 49:498–506.
107. Morscher, E. 1968. "Strength and morphology of growth cartilage under hormonal influence of puberty." *Reconstruc. Sur. Traum.* 10:3–104.
108. Nachemson, A., and Bjure, J. 1973. "The future for the patient with nontreated scoliosis." In *Operative Treatment of Scoliosis.* G. Chapchal, ed. Stuttgart: Thieme, pp. 4–8.

109. ———, and Sahlshand, T. 1977. "Etiologic factors in adolescent idiopathic scoliosis." *Spine* 2:176–184.
110. Nathan, L., and Kuhns, J. G. 1940. "Epiphysitis of the spine." *J. Bone Jt. Surg.* 22:55–62.
111. National Center for Health Statistics. 1978. Health Interview Survey. Unpublished data.
112. Nordwall, A., and Waldenström, J. 1976. "Metachromasia of fibroblasts from patients with idiopathic scoliosis." *Spine* 1:97–98.
113. ———, and Willner, S. 1975. "A study of skeletal age and height in girls with idiopathic scoliosis." *Clin. Orthop.* 110:6–10.
114. Ogden, J. A., and Southwick, W. O. 1976. "Osgood-Schlatter's disease and tibial tuberosity development." *Clin. Orthop.* 116:180–189.
115. ———, and Southwick, W. O. 1977. "Endocrine dysfunction and slipped capital femoral epiphysis." *Yale J. Biol. Med.* 50(1):1–16.
116. Olsen, G. A., Rosen, H., Hohn, R. B., and Slocum, B. 1977. "Electrical muscle stimulation as a means of correcting induced canine scoliotic curves." *Clin. Orthop.* 125:227–235.
117. Pedrini, V. A., Ponseti, I. V., and Dohrman, S. C. 1973. "Glycosaminoglycans of intervertebral disc in idiopathic scoliosis." *J. Lab. Clin. Med.* 82:938–950.
118. Ponseti, I. V., and McClintock, R. 1956. "The pathology of slipping of the upper femoral epiphysis." *J. Bone Jt. Surg. (Amer.)* 38:71–83.
119. Ratliff, A. M. C. 1968. "Traumatic separation of the upper femoral epiphysis in young children." *J. Bone Jt. Surg. (Brit.)* 50:757–770.
120. Reichelt, A., and Rutt, A. 1969. "Untersuchgen zur atiologie der epiphysiolysis bzw. Epiphysiolisthesis capitis femoris." *Arch. Orthop. Unfallchir.* 67:28–38.
121. Rennie, A. M. 1967. "Familial slipped upper femoral epiphysis." *J. Bone Jt. Surg. (Brit.)* 49:535–539.
122. ———, and Mitchell, N. 1974. "Slipped capital femoral epiphysis occurring during growth hormone treatment." *J. Bone Jt. Surg. (Brit.)* 56:703–705.
123. Resnick, D., and Niwayama, G. 1978. "Intravertebral disk herniations: cartilaginous (Schmorl's) nodes." *Radiology* 126:57–65.
124. Reynolds, E. L., and Songtag, L. W. 1944. "Seasonal variation in weight, height, and appearance of ossification centers." *J. Pediatrics* 24:524–535.
125. Riddle, H. F., and Roaf, R. 1955. "Imbalance in the causation of scoliosis." *Lancet* 2:1245.
126. Riseborough, E. J., Wynne-Davies, R. 1973. "A genetic survey of idiopathic scoliosis in Boston, Massachusetts." *J. Bone Jt. Surg. (Amer.)* 55:974–982.
127. Risser, J. L. 1964. "Scoliosis: Past and present." *J. Bone Jt. Surg. (Amer.)* 46:167–199.
128. Robin, G. C., and Cohen, T. 1975. "Familial scoliosis: A clinical report." *J. Bone Jt. Surg. (Brit.)* 57:146–148.
129. Rogala, E. J., Drummond, D. S., and Gurr, J. 1978. "Scoliosis: Incidence and natural history, a prospective epidemiological study." *J. Bone Jt. Surg. (Amer.)* 60:173–176.
130. Sahlstrand, T. 1980. "An analysis of lateral predominance in adolescent idiopathic scoliosis with special reference to convexity of the curve." *Spine* 5:512–518.
131. ———, Örtengren, R., and Nachemson, A. 1978. "Postural equilibrium in adolescent idiopathic scoliosis." *Acta Orthop. Scand.* 49:354–365.
132. ———, Petruson, B., and Örtengren, R., 1979. "Vestibulospinal reflexactivity in patients with adolescent idiopathic scoliosis." *Acta Orthop. Scand.* 50:275–281.
133. Schaefer, R. L., and Purcell, F. H. 1941. "Juvenile osteochondreal (chondroepiphysitis) hypothyroidism." *Amer. J. Surg.* 54:589–604.

134. Scheuermann, H. W. 1921. "Kyphosis dorsalis juvenilis." *Z. Orthop. Chir.* 41:305, as reprinted in *Clin. Orthop.* 128:5–7, 1977.
135. Schmorl, G., and Junghanns, H. 1971. *The Human Spine in Health and Disease,* New York: Grune and Stratton, pp. 158–172, 345–354.
136. Segil, C. M. 1974. "The incidence of idiopathic scoliosis in the Bantu and white population groups in Johannesburg." *J. Bone Jt. Surg. (Brit.)* 56:393.
137. Shands, A. R., and Eisberg, H. B. 1955. "The incidence of scoliosis in the state of Delaware." *J. Bone Jt. Surg. (Amer.)* 37:1243–1249.
138. Smyrnis, P., Valavanis, J., Alexopoulos, A., Siderakis, G., and Giannestras, N. J. 1979. "School screening for scoliosis in Athens." *J. Bone Jt. Surg. (Brit.)* 61:215–217.
139. Sørenson, K. H. 1968. "Slipped upper femoral epiphysis." *Acta Orthop. Scand.* 39:499–517.
140. Span, Y., Robin, G., and Makin, M. 1976. "Incidence of scoliosis in school children in Jerusalem." *J. Bone Jt. Surg. (Brit.)* 58:379.
141. Spencer, G. S. G., and Eccles, M. J. 1976. "Spinal muscle in scoliosis. Part 2: The proportion and size of type 1 and type 2 skeletal muscle fibres measured using a computer-controlled microscope." *J. Neurol. Sci.* 30:143–154.
142. ———, and Zorab, P. A. 1976. "Spinal muscle in scoliosis comparison of normal and scoliotic rabbits." *J. Neurol. Sci.* 30:405–410.
143. Stoddard, A., and Osborn, J. F. 1979. "Scheuermann's disease or spinal osteochondrosis." *J. Bone Jt. Surg. (Brit.)* 61:56–58.
144. Tanner, J. M. 1962. *Growth at Adolescence.* Oxford: Blackwell.
145. Trontelj, J. V., Pecak, F., and Dimitrijevie, M. R. 1979. "Segmental neurophysiological mechanisms in scoliosis." *J. Bone Jt. Surg. (Brit.)* 61:310–313.
146. Wansbrough, R. M., Carrie, A. W., Waler, N. F., and Ruckerbauer, G. 1959. "Coxa plana: its genetic aspects and results of treatment with long Taylor walking caliper: Long-term follow-up study." *J. Bone Jt. Surg. (Amer.)* 41:135–146.
147. Wardle, E. N. 1933. "Etiology and treatment of slipped epiphysis of the head of the femur." *Brit. J. Surg.* 21:313–328.
148. Wassmann, K. 1951. "Kyphosis juvenilis Scheuermann—An occupational disorder." *Acta Orthop. Scand.* 21:65–74.
149. White, A. A., and Panjabi, M. M. 1978. *The Clinical Biomechanics of the Spine.* Philadelphia: Lippincott.
150. ———, Panjabi, M. M., and Thomas, C. C. 1977. "The clinical biomechanics of kyphotic deformities." *Clin. Orthop.* 128:8–17.
151. Willner, P. 1969. "Osgood-Schlatter's disease: Etiology and treatment." *Clin. Orthop.* 62:178–179.
152. Willner, S. 1974. "Growth in height of children with scoliosis." *Acta Orthop. Scand.* 45:854–866.
153. ———. 1974. "A study of growth in girls with adolescent idiopathic structural scoliosis." *Clin. Orthop* 101:129–135.
154. ———. 1975. "The proportion of legs to trunk in girls with idiopathic structural scoliosis." *Acta Orthop. Scand.* 46:84–89.
155. ———. 1975. "A study of height, weight, and menarche in girls with idiopathic structural scoliosis." *Acta Orthop. Scand.* 46:71–83.
156. ———, Nilsson, K. O., Kastrup, K., and Beigstrand, G. G. 1976. "Growth hormone and somatomedin A in girls with adolescent idiopathic scoliosis." *Acta Paediat. Scand.* 65:547–552.
157. Wilson, P. D., Jacobs, B., and Schecter, L. 1965. "Slipped capital femoral epiphysis." *J. Bone Jt. Surg. (Amer.)* 47:1128–1145.

158. Winter, R. B. 1978. "The Spine." In *Pediatric Orthopaedics*. W. W. Lovell and R. B. Winter, eds. Philadelphia: Lippincott, pp. 573–684.
159. Woolfrey, B. F., and Chandler, E. F. 1960. "Manifestations of Osgood-Schlatter's disease in late teenage and early adulthood." *J. Bone Jt. Surg. (Amer.)* 42:327–332.
160. Wynne-Davies, R. 1968. "Familial (idiopathic) scoliosis. A family survey." *J. Bone Jt. Surg. (Brit.)* 50:24–30.
161. ———, and Gormley, J. 1978. "The aetiology of Perthes disease." *J. Bone Jt. Surg. (Brit.)* 60:6–14.
162. Yamada, K., Yamamoto, H., Ikata, T., Nakagawa, Y., Kinoshita, I., Tezuka, A., and Tamura, T. 1971. "A neurological approach to the etiology and therapy of scoliosis." *J. Bone Jt. Surg. (Amer.)* 53:197.
163. ———, Yamamoto, H., Tamura, T., and Tezuka, A. 1974. "Development of scoliosis under neurological basis, particularly in relation with brain-stem abnormalities." *J. Bone Jt. Surg. (Amer.)* 56:1764–1765.
164. Zuk, T. 1962. "The role of spinal abdominal muscles in the pathogenesis of scoliosis." *J. Bone Jt. Surg. (Brit.)* 44:102–105.

4 The Arthritic Disorders

Among the many types of arthritic disorders, or joint diseases, osteoarthrosis and rheumatoid arthritis are by far the most common in Western populations. Gout, ankylosing spondylitis, and juvenile rheumatoid arthritis are also considered in this chapter, although they occur less frequently. According to the United States Health Interview Survey, about 10 percent of the population of all ages report that they have suffered from arthritis during the preceding year and that they have sought medical care for it or have had to limit their activity because of it (228). Almost one-quarter of these people feel they are "affected all the time" by arthritis and rheumatism.

The arthritic disorders may be grouped into the following four categories: (1) osteoarthrosis, which generally occurs as a result of changes related to aging and wear and tear on joints, (2) joint diseases caused by some more general pathologic process, such as gout, which is closely related to high concentrations of serum uric acid resulting from abnormal purine metabolism, (3) joint diseases thought to be related to disorders of the immune system, such as rheumatoid arthritis, juvenile rheumatoid arthritis, and ankylosing spondylitis, and (4) forms of arthritis caused by specific microorganisms; these will not be considered here.

Much of the recent research on rheumatoid arthritis, juvenile rheumatoid arthritis, and especially ankylosing spondylotis has centered on the HLA system (H standing for human or histocompatibility, L for leucocyte, the cell type first studied, and A for the first system so described) (44). HLA histocompatibility antigens are genetically determined isoantigens present on the vast majority of human cell membranes. They elicit an immune response when grafted to a genetically disparate individual and thus determine the compatibility of tissues in transplantation (41). The loci for the HLA system are located on the sixth chromosome; four of these loci have been described to date: HLA-A, HLA-B, HLA-C, and HLA-D. Every individual has a paternal and a maternal chromosome, each bearing the four corresponding HLA alleles. Thus, each individual may have two antigenic specificities for each of the four loci; the specificities of these surface antigens have been assigned numbers (e.g., HLA-A1, HLA-B27). Since several possible specificities exist for each loci, there are numerous combinations that occur, and the probability of any two randomly selected individuals having completely identical specificities is low.

Antigens encoded by the HLA-A and HLA-B loci most readily evoke the formation of complement-fixing cytotoxic antibodies that can be used for tissue typing; HLA-C induces a weaker response (264). The precise antigenic identities for HLA-A, HLA-B, and HLA-C are determined using panels of donor lymphocytes of known antigenicity along with specific antisera. The fourth locus, HLA-D, which carries genes involved with lymphocytic-activating determinants, is more difficult to type directly. Because the HLA-D locus is closely linked and perhaps identical to a locus called HLA-DR, and because HLA-DR antigens may be detected on B lymphocytes, HLA-D specificities are at present detected indirectly using panels of donor B lymphocytes. The letter w following a locus symbol and preceding a specificity number indicates that a specificity is still provisionally identified (44).

Interest in the relationship between certain arthritic disorders and the HLA system stems from the belief that these diseases have an autoimmune etiology and from the observation that the chromosomal locus governing the histocompatibility antigens is linked to immune response genes in the mouse. One particular histocompatibility antigen, HLA-B27, has been found in a much higher proportion of patients with ankylosing spondylitis, Reiter's syndrome, and spondylitis associated inflammatory bowel disease and psoriasis than in the general population. The most common disease in this group of spondyloarthropathies is ankylosing spondylitis, which will be discussed later in this chapter together with possible explanations of its association with HLA-B27. Some evidence exists for a weaker association of rheumatoid arthritis with HLA-DR and HLA-D antigens, while for juvenile rheumatoid arthritis an initially reported association with HLA-B27 was found to be accounted for by the children who went on to develop ankylosing spondylitis (97).

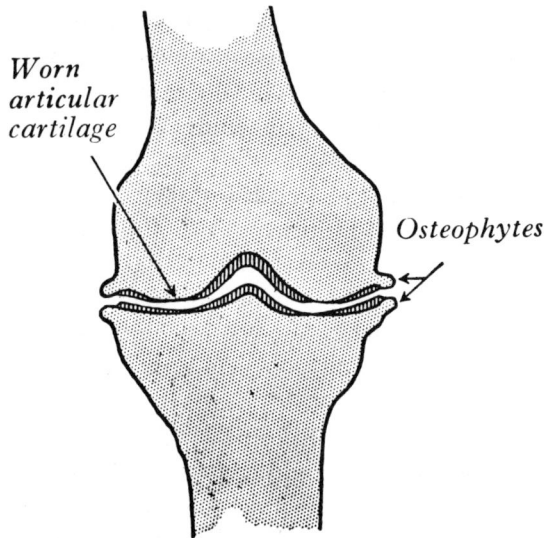

Figure 4-1 Osteoarthrosis.

Source: Adams (8).

OSTEOARTHROSIS

Osteoarthrosis, also called osteoarthritis or degenerative joint disease, is the most frequently occurring joint disease. The articular cartilage of diarthrodial joints becomes roughened, eroded, and thin, and the bone underneath the affected cartilage thickens (subchondral bone sclerosis). Cysts may form beneath the sclerosed bone, and the cartilage at the edges of the articular plate grows outward (marginal lipping). As the disease progresses, the cartilage at the edges becomes calcified and ossified. The spurs of bone thus formed are called osteophytes, and are characteristic of advanced osteoarthrosis (see Figure 4-1).

One or several joints may be affected. The usual initial symptoms are pain in the joint and stiffness after periods of inactivity; then, the pain and stiffness may become continuous, with restriction of movement and sometimes joint deformity. Diagnosis is made by X-ray, which, in early stages of the disease, shows narrowing of the joint space corresponding to the thinning of the articular cartilage. In later stages sclerosis of subchrondral bone and osteophytes may be observed. For epidemiologic surveys, the *Atlas of Standard Radiographs of Arthritis* has been published (309) in which four grades (doubtful, minimal, moderate, severe) are illustrated by a series of photographs considered to show the characteristic stages through which the disease progresses in various joints. This has, to some extent, made possible comparisons of the results of different surveys, although considerable observer variability still exists (170,335).

Frequency and Demographic Characteristics

Table 4-1 shows prevalence rates of osteoarthrosis of the hands and feet as determined from X-rays taken in a probability sample of the population of ages 18 to 79 years in the United States (225). Prevalence rates in these joints, as in all joints, increase markedly with age. While only 7.2 percent of males and 1.6 percent of females of 18 to 24 years of age show X-ray evidence of osteoarthrosis in their hands and feet, almost everyone in the 75 to 79 year group has X-ray evidence of osteoarthrosis. In this survey as well as others (6,171,194,218), males have been found to be affected more frequently than females below about 45 years of age, whereas above this age females are afflicted more frequently and more severely than males. The joints most often found on X-ray to have moderate or severe osteoarthrosis are indicated in Table 4-2 (171). Clearly, males and females differ with respect to the types of joints affected, probably reflecting both variation between the sexes in the joints most subject to stress and the higher prevalence of generalized osteoarthrosis in females than in males.

Many people with radiographic evidence of osteoarthrosis, however,

Table 4-1   Prevalence, in Percent, of X-ray Evidence of Osteoarthrosis of the Hands and/or Feet in Adults Aged 18–79 Years, by Age and Sex, United States, 1960–1962

	Age (years)	Males	Females
	18–24	7.2	1.6
	25–34	13.6	6.2
	35–44	30.2	19.6
	45–54	47.0	46.3
	55–64	63.2	75.2
	65–74	75.8	84.7
	75–79	80.9	89.8
Total	18–79	37.4	37.3

Source: National Center for Health Statistics (225).

Table 4-2   Prevalence, in Percent, of X-ray Evidence of Moderate and Severe Osteoarthrosis in Leigh, England, in the Age Group 55–64 by Sex and Joint

Joint		Males	Females
Distal interphalangeal	Hands	11.0	17.0
Proximal interphalangeal		2.3	12.1
Metacarpophalangeal		6.4	1.5
First carpometacarpal		6.4	16.0
Wrists		1.7	0
Cervical spine		3.5	3.0
Lumbar spine		7.9	7.3
Hips		8.4	3.1
Sacroiliac		1.2	1.6
Knees		11.1	15.1
Tarsi		1.2	2.9
Lateral metatarsophalangeal	Feet	0	1.0
First metatarsophalangeal		8.7	17.5
Total		43.4	46.9

Source: J. H. Kellgren and J. S. Lawrence (171).

have no symptoms or disability. For instance, in a British survey of miners and men in other occupational groups (168), only one-fourth of those with X-ray evidence of osteoarthrosis in the knee gave a history of pain in their knee. Recent data from the U.S. Health and Nutrition Examination Survey (227) indicate that only 57 percent of people with evidence of severe osteoarthrosis of the hip reported significant hip pain on most days for at least one month. Although there is a definite relationship between extent of symptoms and X-ray findings (194,227), it is not known why some people with X-ray changes have symptoms while others do not. It has been found that subjective and objective indicators of osteoarthrosis are more strongly correlated in women than in men (4,5,7). Although such data have been used as evidence that women complain more than men (5), they may also be interpreted as indicating that men tend to deny symptoms more often than do women. More research on these relationships is required.

Generalized Osteoarthrosis

Osteoarthrosis may involve individual joints because of particular stresses on those joints, or may occur in the form of generalized osteoarthrosis, which is less closely related to particular stresses on joints and which affects females more frequently than males. Although it is impossible to separate with certainty all cases of generalized osteoarthrosis from all other cases, in generalized osteoarthrosis the distal interphalangeal joints of fingers are characteristically affected along with several other joints of the body, particularly the first carpometacarpal joints, the first tarso-metatarsal joints, the metatarsophalangeal joints of the great toe, the interfacetal joints of the cervical and lumbar spine, and the knees (165,171,173). There are said to be both nodal and nonnodal forms of generalized osteoarthrosis (172,192), the nodal form referring to the presence of Heberden's nodes, which are bony protuberances on the margins of the distal interphalangeal joints. Generalized osteoarthrosis associated with Heberden's nodes is usually the more severe form (172).

The etiologies of these forms of generalized osteoarthrosis have not been well studied. However, it is generally felt that heredity or some general constitutional factor predisposes to generalized osteoarthrosis, particularly to the nodal form (165,171,173,304). Also, previous inflammatory seronegative polyarthritis and hyperuricemia appear to be associated with the nonnodal form (172,192).

Geographic Variation

Although X-ray-determined prevalence rates of osteoarthrosis are relatively uniform in different Western Caucasian populations, in other parts of the world there are populations with particularly high or low prevalence rates in specific joints. Osteoarthrosis of the hip, for instance, is rarely seen in Chinese (147). Hypothesized explanations for this are a low prevalence of predisposing hip disorders in Chinese (147) and a tendency of Chinese to squat rather than to sit (126); in a squatting position all areas of the articular cartilage are subject to pressure relatively evenly. Osteoarthrosis of the knees is more common in women on the west coast than on the east coast of Greenland. It has been postulated that the occupational stresses on the knees of women on the west coast, who usually work outside the home, are responsible for their higher rates (15). Low prevalence rates of osteoarthrosis of the metatarsophalangeal joint in Jamaicans and in black South Africans have been attributed to their walking without shoes (50,295). Higher than expected prevalence rates of osteoarthrosis of the knees among Jamaicans have been thought to be related to the rough footpaths over which they walk (50).

Suggested Etiologic Agents

Other than the aging process itself, wear and tear on joints is generally considered to be the most important etiologic factor for osteoarthrosis of specific joints. Epidemiologic evidence comes from various sources. Prevalence studies carried out in specific occupational groups have shown that miners have high prevalence rates of osteoarthrosis of the elbows and knees (187), cotton pickers have high rates of osteoarthrosis of the fingers (190), and dockers have an excess of osteoarthrosis of the fingers, elbows, and knees (247). In the New Haven Survey of Joint Diseases, it was found that the right hand was affected more frequently and more severely than the left, especially in right-handed people, suggesting that perhaps minor trauma from repetitive tasks predisposes to osteoarthrosis (4). In addition, more osteoarthrosis is found in the stronger than in the weaker leg of people with previous poliomyelitis (119). Other associations of specific activities with osteoarthrosis of specific sites have been reviewed by Lee et al. (197), although most are based on small numbers or on anecdotal information. These associations include osteoarthrosis of the ankles, feet, and knees in soccer players; osteoarthrosis of the knees in American football players; osteoarthrosis of the hands in boxers; osteoarthrosis of the ankles and feet in ballet dancers; osteoarthrosis of the shoulders and elbows in baseball pitchers; osteoarthrosis of the patellar-femoral joint in cyclists, osteoarthrosis of the fingers in cricket bowlers; osteoarthrosis of the ankles and knees in lacrosse players; and osteoarthrosis of the spine, knees, and elbows in wrestlers. In contrast, X-rays of the hips of competitive runners do not indicate an excess of osteoarthrotic changes; the investigators who reported this finding point out that the hip joint is made for motion, and that stress from running should not be detrimental to the joint (256).

Thus, although the evidence is persuasive that wear and tear contribute to the development of osteoarthrosis in a variety of joints, the specific types of wear and tear that predispose to this disease are not known; it is likely that some types of mechanical stress predispose to osteoarthrosis while other types do not. For instance, it is not known whether the high risk for osteoarthrosis of the knees in miners is attributable to multiple injuries, frequent twisting, or some other specific motion.

Other established risk factors for osteoarthrosis of specific joints are previous diseases affecting the joint, faulty body mechanics, or single episodes such as fractures that occur through a joint or that result in malalignment of the joint. In the hip joint, for instance, congenital dislocation of the hip, Legg-Calvé-Perthes disease, or slipped epiphysis can lead to the development of osteoarthrosis of the hip in the early adult years. At the knee joint, ligamentous instability, loose bodies, and torn cartilages predispose to osteoarthrosis. Degeneration of intervertebral discs (103,158), spondylolisthesis (171,204), and lumbosacral transitional vertebrae (219) each may increase the likelihood that osteoarthrosis will develop in the lumbar spine. Similar conditions predispose to osteoarthrosis in other joints. Even minor abnormalities may be responsible for incongruities of articulation in joints, which in turn may lead to premature degenerative changes (224). Prevalence studies in which questions have been asked about previous joint symptoms (192) and in which antistreptolysin 0 titers have been measured (6) have suggested that subclinical polyarthritis may also predispose to osteoarthrosis, particularly generalized osteoarthrosis.

Obesity has received attention in several studies. It has been shown that generalized osteoarthrosis as well as osteoarthrosis of the hands and feet are more common in obese people (6,102,171). However, the evidence has been contradictory as to whether obesity predisposes to osteoarthrosis of the large weight-bearing joints such as the hip and knee joints (6,171,196,275). One possible reason for the discrepant findings is that people with osteoarthrosis in these joints reduce their activity, so that it is difficult to know whether osteoarthrosis causes obesity or whether obesity causes osteoarthrosis. Some evidence from animal studies suggests that diet may be involved in the etiology of osteoarthrosis rather than obesity per se (289,294).

Summary

The strongest risk factor for osteoarthrosis is age; indeed, this disorder seems to be an almost inevitable consequence of aging. Nonetheless, osteoarthrosis occurs earlier and more severely in some people than in others, and may be generalized or localized. Wear and tear undoubtedly contribute to the development of osteoarthrosis in specific joints, but it is not clear exactly what types of wear and tear are most detrimental. Previous joint disorders are known to increase the risk for osteoarthrosis of specific joints, but further study is needed to determine whether subclinical polyarthritis is a risk factor for generalized osteoarthrosis. Relatively little is known about risk factors for generalized osteoarthrosis, except that heredity probably is involved. The association of generalized osteoarthrosis with obesity suggests an etiologic role of some general metabolic process. In trying to learn more about the etiology of osteoarthrosis of any joint, it would be helpful to consider generalized osteoarthrosis separately from localized osteoarthrosis. Finally, it will be important to learn more about why some people with a given degree of X-ray change have more symptoms and disability than others, since it is the symptoms and disability that make osteoarthrosis such an important disease.

RHEUMATOID ARTHRITIS

Rheumatoid arthritis is a systemic disease primarily affecting the connective tissue surrounding joints; occasionally connective tissue in other organs such as the heart may be involved as well. Although in early stages only one joint may be affected, the disease generally progresses rapidly to other joints. Typically, the small joints of the hands and feet are affected first, followed by the elbows, knees, shoulders, and hips. Joint involvement is usually symmetrical. In severe cases, joints throughout the body may be involved. Since rheumatoid arthritis is a systemic disease, loss of appetite, weight loss, general malaise, and depression may accompany the joint changes.

Within the joints, inflammatory changes are seen in the synovial membranes and articular structures, and fluid may accumulate in the joints. The usual symptoms are pain and morning stiffness. The joints and surrounding tendons, ligaments, and joint capsules are tender and swollen. If the inflammatory process continues, damage to the joint cartilage, tendons, subchondral bone , and other surrounding structures occurs. In the hands of the rheumatoid arthritic, the proximal interphalangeal and metacarpophalangeal joints are typically swollen, and, as the disease progresses, the metacarpophalangeal joints are deviated to the ulnar side. The appearance of a hand of a typical rheumatoid arthritic is shown in Figure 4-2.

Rheumatoid arthritis has a variable course. Among patients seen at hospitals or clinics, the disease is generally characterized by periods of remission and exacerbation, but the overall course tends to be slow and relentless, with the affected joints left permanently damaged. In a six-year follow-up study of patients who had been admitted to a hospital with rheumatoid arthritis, for instance, only 24 percent were able to carry on

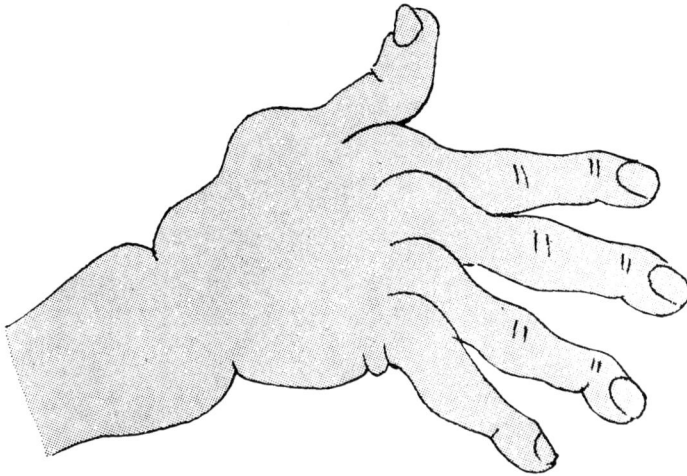

Figure 4-2   Typical appearance of rheumatoid arthritis in the hand.
Source: Aston (26).

all normal activities; 40 percent were moderately incapacitated, 26 percent were more severely crippled, and 10 percent had become helpless and dependent on others (93). Generalizations cannot be made from cases seen at medical care facilities (10), however, and population-based studies indicate a much broader spectrum of disease severity, including some transient cases that do not leave any permanent evidence of deformity. It is not known whether these transient cases really are rheumatoid arthritis (215).

In addition to the pain and limitation of activity associated with many cases, the psychological effects may be serious, since from the early stages of the disease there is considerable anxiety about the possibility of crippling and about the appearance of the hands (98). Mortality rates among rheumatoid arthritics are higher than in the general population; the excess mortality is attributable mostly to infectious diseases, especially of the respiratory tract (12,152,221,320).

Despite the severe course that rheumatoid arthritis often takes, the relatively large number of studies that have been undertaken of its causation, and the strong likelihood that autoimmunity is involved in its etiology, the actual causes are unknown. Many of the epidemiologic studies

Table 4-3 Summary of Diagnostic Criteria for Rheumatoid Arthritis

Classical Rheumatoid Arthritis
  Seven of the following criteria are required:
  1. Morning stiffness for at least six weeks.
  2. Pain on motion or tenderness in at least one joint for at least six weeks.
  3. Swelling in at least one joint for at least six weeks.
  4. Swelling of at least one other joint for at least six weeks.
  5. Symmetrical joint swelling with simultaneous involvement of the same joint on both sides of the body for at least six weeks. Terminal phalangeal joint involvement will not satisfy this criterion.
  6. Subcutaneous nodules.
  7. X-ray changes typical of rheumatoid arthritis.
  8. Demonstration of rheumatoid factor or positive streptococcal agglutination test.
  9. Poor mucin precipitate from synovial fluid.
  10. Characteristic histologic changes in synovial membrane with three or more of the following: marked villous hypertrophy; proliferation of superficial synovial cells often with palisading; marked infiltration of chronic inflammatory cells with tendency to form "lymphoid nodules"; deposition of compact fibrin, either on surface or interstitially; foci of cell necrosis.
  11. Characteristic histologic changes in nodules showing granulomatous foci with central zones of cell necrosis, surrounded by proliferated fixed cells, and peripheral fibrosis and chronic inflammatory cell infiltration, predominantly perivascular.

Definite Rheumatoid Arthritis
  Five of the criteria listed under "classical rheumatoid arthritis" must be satisfied.

Probable Rheumatoid Arthritis
  Three of the criteria listed under "classical rheumatoid arthritis" must be satisfied.

Possible Rheumatoid Arthritis
  Two of the following criteria must be satisfied and total duration of joint symptoms must be at least three weeks:
  1. Morning stiffness.
  2. Tenderness or pain on motion.
  3. History or observation of joint swelling.
  4. Subcutaneous nodules.
  5. Elevated sedimentation rate or C-reactive protein.
  6. Iritis.

Exclusions
  The presence of any of the following will exclude an individual from the classical, definite, probable, or possible group:
  1. The typical rash of disseminated lupus erythematosus.
  2. High concentration of lupus erythematosus cells.
  3. Histologic evidence of periarteritis nodosa.
  4. Weakness of neck, trunk, and pharyngeal muscles or persistent muscle swelling or dermatomyositis.
  5. Definite scleroderma.
  6. A clinical picture characteristic of rheumatic fever.
  7. A clinical picture characteristic of gouty arthritis.

Table 4-3 (cont.)

8. Tophi.
9. A clinical picture characteristic of acute infectious arthritis of bacterial or viral origin.
10. Tubercule bacilli in the joints or histological evidence of joint tuberculosis.
11. A clinical picture characteristic of Reiter's syndrome.
12. A clinical picture characteristic of the shoulder-hand syndrome.
13. A clinical picture characteristic of hypertrophic pulmonary osteoarthropathy.
14. A clinical picture characteristic of neuroarthropathy.
15. Homogentisic acid in the urine detectable grossly with alkalinization.
16. Histological evidence of sarcoid or positive Kveim test.
17. Multiple myeloma.
18. Characteristic skin lesions of erythema nodosum.
19. Leukemia or lymphoma.
20. Agammaglobulinemia.

Source: Ropes et al. (266).

have had serious methodological limitations, which are discussed in detail by Weiner (327). For instance, diagnostic criteria have posed problems over the years, and it has been pointed out (11) that "typical patients" are rare. Because of the variability in the mode of onset, the joints involved, and the course of the disease, some investigators (74,191,249,327) have speculated that rheumatoid arthritis consists of several distinct disorders. Whether this is so remains to be seen, but in any event, diagnosis may be difficult, especially in the early stages of the disease. The American Rheumatism Association's diagnostic criteria for rheumatoid arthritis (266) have been used in most of the recent epidemiologic studies, and are listed in Table 4-3. Unfortunately, not all investigators have used these criteria in the same way. Also, since their promulgation, their validity and reliability have been debated, but these arguments will not be discussed here.

One of the components of the diagnostic criteria is rheumatoid factor. Rheumatoid factors are antibodies directed against a patient's own gammaglobulins. They are found in the blood of about 2 to 5 percent of the general population, and of about 10 to 25 percent of clinically diagnosed cases of rheumatoid arthritis; the magnitude of these percentages depends considerably on the age and racial group, the geographic area under consideration, and the specific test and diagnostic criteria used (226,321,322). Within a given subgroup of the population, however, the higher the concentration of rheumatoid factors, the greater the likelihood of disease occurrence (327). Also, the course of disease appears to be more severe in cases who are seropositive (69).

Frequency and Demographic Characteristics

In the Health Examination Survey of the National Center for Health Statistics (226), 3.2 percent of the population of ages 18 to 79 years were found to have classical, definite, or probable rheumatoid arthritis; this included 4.6 percent of females and 1.7 percent of males. Table 4-4 shows that prevalence rates increase with age in both sexes. Most studies have found that females are affected three times more frequently than males (68,75,169,189,195,216), although there is some variation probably attributable at least in part to misclassification of cases (333). The ratio of affected females to males appears to be nearer unity for cases in which the onset is after 65 years of age (163,206). The onset of most cases, however, occurs in the age range 20 to 60 years, although the actual peak varies from one study to another and appears to depend on the diagnostic criteria used (206).

Recently, the incidence rates for people seeking medical care for rheumatoid arthritis were determined over a twenty-five year period in the Rochester, Minnesota, area (202). Age-adjusted annual incidence rates were 68.1 per 100,000 for females and 32.6 per 100,000 for males for probable, definite, or classical cases of rheumatoid arthritis. It was also noted that females had incidence rates ranging from around 70 per 100,000 to 90 per 100,000 from 1950 to 1965, which then declined to 40

Table 4-4   Prevalence, in Percent, of Classical, Definite, and Probable Rheumatoid Arthritis in Persons Aged 18–79 Years, by Sex and Age, United States, 1960–1962

Age (years)	Male	Female	Both sexes
18–24	0.2	0.3	0.3
25–34	—	0.6	0.3
35–44	0.5	2.1	1.3
45–54	1.5	4.4	3.0
55–64	4.2	8.3	6.3
65–74	3.1	14.1	9.2
75–79	14.1	23.5	18.8
Total (18–79)	1.7	4.6	3.2

Source: National Center for Health Statistics (226).

per 100,000 from 1970 to 1974. In males, incidence rates had been relatively constant over the entire time period.

Prevalence rates do not appear to be affected by the number of children women have had (191), although some reports suggest that never-married women have less rheumatoid arthritis than expected (75). The divorce rate is high among patients with rheumatoid arthritis (181,209,263), but this is in all likelihood a consequence of the disease, not a cause. With some exceptions (74), most studies indicate that age- and sex-specific prevalence rates are approximately equal in blacks and whites (57,206). Results have been conflicting as to whether rates are higher in urban than in rural areas (74,191,211,296), but this may vary from one geographic area to another. Although some studies have reported no social class differences, most have found prevalence rates to be higher in lower classes (74,181,191). Certain occupational groups have been reported to have somewhat higher-than-expected prevalence rates (74,191), but no consistent patterns have been noticed; it is not certain that the occupations with the highest prevalence rates are indicative of those in which the disease developed.

Rheumatoid arthritis occurs throughout the world (321). Climate, geography, latitude, and altitude do not appear to influence its prevalence. Certain population groups such as the Pima Indians in Arizona (238) and female Yakima Indians of central Washington State (32) have higher than average prevalence rates and Jamaicans have high rates of mild erosive arthritis (193). Other groups such as rural blacks in South Africa (36), Japanese in Japan (288), residents of Jerusalem (9), and Puerto Ricans (210) appear to have low rates, but no explanation has been found for these differences. The Pima Indians have an especially high prevalence of rheumatoid factor, but the reasons for this are again not known (238). Although methodological and observer variation may account for some of these differences, such as the low rates in Puerto Rico and Japan (74), many of the differences are likely to be real since the same investigators were involved in some of the studies in different locations. In Jerusalem the prevalence is found to be higher among immigrants from Europe than among those from North Africa or Asia (9).

Suggested Etiologic Agents

Other than the higher prevalence rates in females than males and the tendency of most cases to be initially diagnosed during early or middle adult years, few aspects of the distribution of rheumatoid arthritis in the population have provided leads to etiology. In fact, many aspects of the descriptive data have been conflicting, probably because of different diagnostic criteria, methods of study, selection of subjects, and populations from which the subjects are chosen. One useful observation is the apparent decrease in incidence rates with time among females in Rochester, Minnesota (202). This has provided some support for the recent finding in a cohort study in England (332) that women who used oral contraceptives had an incidence rate of rheumatoid arthritis that was half of that among nonusers. An earlier study (118) had also provided some evidence of lower-than-expected numbers of cases among women using oral contraceptives. These results, although needing further verification, are consistent with the frequently made observation that many women have remission of symptoms during pregnancy (57). It is felt that the remission of symptoms during pregnancy is attributable to altered immunologic function by some unknown mechanism (57).

The possibility that heredity is involved in the etiology of rheumatoid arthritis has interested investigators for many years, and numerous studies of rheumatoid arthritis in families have been reported. O'Brien (237), in 1967, extensively reviewed seventeen family studies and several twin studies and concluded that there was little evidence for familial clustering in rheumatoid arthritis, and that many of the studies showing a genetic predisposition had serious methodological flaws. Since then, studies of the frequency of occurrence of human leukocyte antigens (HLA) in patients with rheumatoid arthritis suggest that there may in fact be an inherited susceptibility. (For a brief description of the HLA system, see pp. 78–79.) Several studies have indicated that adult Caucasian rheumatoid arthritis patients have an increased prevalence of HLA-DRw4 and of HLA-Dw4 relative to normal controls (91,117,154,246,300,313). These studies generally indicate that persons with the DRw4 and Dw4 antigens have about six times the risk of developing rheumatoid arthritis as those without these histocompatibility antigens. In blacks, the association between rheumatoid arthritis and these antigens does not appear to be so strong (300). Except for a Japanese study that showed a high frequency of Bw22 among rheumatoid arthritis patients (316), no associations between rheumatoid arthritis and HLA at the A, B, or C locus have been demonstrated. Two other D-locus antigens (DRw2 and DRw1) have been found to occur less frequently than expected among patients with rheumatoid arthritis (117,246,313). Although higher than expected frequencies of Dw4 and DRw4 in affected members of families in which related individuals have rheumatoid arthritis (154,177) and of DRw4 in patients with family histories of rheumatoid arthritis have been reported (246), other studies have not found DRw4 to be in excess in affected family members (37).

These observed associations of HLA-DRw4 and HLA-Dw4 with rheumatoid arthritis are generally believed to indicate an inherited susceptibility to the disease. The D locus is not considered to be directly involved, but rather it is felt to be linked to one or more immune response genes that have a more direct role in disease pathogenesis.

Indeed, many investigators feel that the joint inflammation and systemic manifestations in rheumatoid arthritis result from a series of immunopathologic or autoimmune responses. Immune complexes consisting of antibodies to IgG (rheumatoid factors) and IgM are considered to be prominent features of the disease; several investigators (245,293,326,329) have reported that rheumatoid factor complexes in the synovial tissue contribute directly to the inflammatory response. The interaction of these complexes with the complement system and possibly with other antigen-antibody complexes such as antinuclear, antilymphocytic, and antithyroglobulin complexes, is believed to result in tissue damage (245). Defective cell-mediated immune response has been found in at least some patients with rheumatoid arthritis (28,89,245,283).

The aberrant immunologic responses seen in patients with rheumatoid arthritis are thought to result from a persistent antigenic stimulus. Although infectious agents have been suspected for some time, little direct evidence exists for an infectious etiology. In general, attempts to isolate viral DNA and RNA from the synovia and lymphocytes of patients with rheumatoid arthritis have not been successful (72,235,236,329). Some evidence indicates that synovial lymphocytes are engaged in a persistent antiviral response and are therefore not able to respond to new infections (25,245,329). Recently, the Epstein-Barr virus (EBV) has received considerable attention as a possible causative agent. Patients with rheumatoid arthritis have a high frequency of antibody to an antigen seen in EBV infected cells, which in turn is closely related to EBV nuclear antigen. Rheumatoid arthritics also exhibit higher titers to anti-EBV nuclear antigen than do controls. Furthermore, EBV is capable of inducing rheumatoid factor production in normal cells (14,88,89,245,292,307). The evidence for an etiologic role of EBV is far from conclusive, however, and other infectious agents have been proposed as well, including bacteria and mycoplasma (40,72,76,249,293,302,307,326,330).

Finally, the role of psychological factors in the development of the disease has long been of interest. Many of the relevant studies have been reviewed critically by Weiner (327), and will not be discussed here. One psychological profile of high-risk individuals that has emerged is of adults who as adolescents were rebellious, aggressive, and tomboyish, and who as adults express this in tyrannical and domineering behavior toward others, or who are controlled by various psychological defense mechanisms or by self-punitive actions, which often lead to suffering. In contrast, others, particularly women, are angry, resentful, and embittered, but try not to express these feelings. Weiner feels that there is somewhat stronger evidence suggesting that separation from another person, especially from someone who has been submissive to the potential case and who has felt trapped in the relationship, may precipitate the onset of the disease. He notes, however, that all such data have been collected retrospectively, and it is difficult to differentiate between those psychological factors that may precipitate rheumatoid arthritis and those that may be consequences of the disease, and that people may not accurately recall the temporal relationship between the putative precipitating event and the disease onset. Also, it is possible (79) that psychologically traumatic events may contribute to a person's decision to seek medical care and thus appear to have precipitated the disease. In any event, definitive evidence on the role of psychological variables in the onset of the disease would require carefully conducted prospective studies.

In summary, it is highly likely that an abnormal immune response plays an important role in the etiology of rheumatoid arthritis. However, the specific agents involved in this immunopathology have not been identified.

JUVENILE RHEUMATOID ARTHRITIS

Juvenile rheumatoid arthritis, called Still's disease in England, is a chronic polyarthritis affecting children, usually accompanied by fever, enlargement of lymph nodes, and enlargement of the spleen. It differs from adult rheumatoid arthritis in several ways: circulating rheumatoid factors are not common; ankylosing spondylitis is a frequent symptom; and iritis, inflammation of the ciliary body, and pathology in the cornea occur more frequently than in the adult form. Although considerable variation occurs in the course of the disease, the prognosis for patients with juvenile rheumatoid arthritis is generally better than for those with the adult form. About 75 percent of the juvenile rheumatoid arthritis patients have long remissions with no permanent joint damage (29,132,234,278).

Criteria for juvenile rheumatoid arthritis were first specified by the American Rheumatism Association in 1973. Revised criteria, established in 1977, defined juvenile rheumatoid arthritis as persistent arthritis in one or more joints for six or more weeks, providing that all exclusion criteria were met. The sixteenth birthday is usually considered to be the upper age limit (206). Three subtypes were described, based upon the type of onset during the first six months of the disease: (1) systemic or Still's type, which is characterized by a persistent high fever and rash and/or organ involvement within the first six months of disease onset, (2) pauciarticular onset, which involves four or fewer joints during the first six months and excludes patients with systemic onset disease, and (3) polyarticular onset, which involves five or more joints within the first six months and also excludes cases with systemic onset type of disease (51). Despite the establishment of these criteria, diagnosis of juvenile rheumatoid arthritis is often difficult. Also, studies that were conducted before the criteria were established or that have not strictly adhered to the criteria have made comparisons among investigations of somewhat limited value. In any event, most information on the characteristics of patients affected with the disease comes from case series, not from population-based studies.

The most frequent time of onset for all three subtypes of juvenile rheumatoid arthritis combined is between 1 and 3 years of age (20,131,140,186,198,234,281,306). A second peak has been reported between the ages of 9 and 14 years (186,206,234,306). Combining all subtypes, females are affected more frequently than males by about 2 to 1 (20,131,140,186,234).

However, these demographic characteristics differ according to subtype. Systemic onset juvenile rheumatoid arthritis, which accounts for about 20 percent of all cases (111,198,206,234,278,280), affects males and females with approximately equal frequency (131,198,206,278,280). The average age at onset is generally reported to be 6 years (111,280,306). Pauciarticular onset disease is observed in about 30 to 40 percent of cases (62,131,151,206), with a mean age of onset of less than 5 years of age and a female predominance. A subgroup of pauciarticular onset cases is HLA B27 positive; these are predominantly males, have a late age at onset, and frequently progress to frank ankylosing spondylitis. The polyarticular mode of onset is seen in 30 to 50 percent of cases (62,198,206,280) with a mean age of onset of 5 to 6 years and a female predominance (111,131,206).

The mode-of-onset subtypes differ in other respects. Patients with the systemic-onset subtype do not show evidence of antinuclear antibodies and rheumatoid factor, and few have inflammation of the iris and ciliary body of the eye (131,198,278–280). The pauciarticular B27 negative group frequently does have antinuclear antibodies, seldom has rheumatoid factor but usually does have inflammation of the iris and ciliary body; also, large joints are generally affected (21,131,198,278–280). In the pauciarticular B27 positive subtype, which often progresses to clinical ankylosing spondylitis, there is usually notable sacroiliac involvement, acute inflammation of the iris and ciliary body, large joint involvement, but no rheumatoid factor or antinuclear antibodies (20,21,278,279). The polyarticular onset subtype is generally found in association with rheumatoid factor, elevated antinuclear antibodies, and small joint involvement (21,131,278–280). Patients with the polyarticular mode of onset with positive rheumatoid factors have the poorest prognosis, as the disease frequently progresses to severe disease with erosive arthritis (67,130,279,280,303). Some patients may in fact have adult rheumatoid arthritis with an early onset.

Because of the different characteristics of the various subtypes of juvenile rheumatoid arthritis, many investigators feel that they represent several distinct diseases, each with its own etiology (21,129,131,206,278–280,306).

Estimates of the overall incidence rate of juvenile rheumatoid arthritis are generally based on cases seeking care at specialty clinics and hospitals. Such estimates of annual incidence rates have ranged from 3 to 9 per 10,000 in persons under 16 years of age in various populations (145,186,306). Prevalence rates have been estimated as 6 per 10,000 over a five-year period in the school population around Taplow, England (59). Other estimates of prevalence have been made by multiplying the known prevalence of adult rheumatoid arthritis by the ratio of the number of cases of juvenile rheumatoid arthritis to the number of cases of adult rheumatoid arthritis; this has led to estimates of prevalence rates ranging from 8 to 48 per 10,000 (31,206).

Blacks in the United States do not appear to have incidence and prevalence rates much different from whites (131,198), although possible differences between rates in blacks and whites have apparently not been studied for individual subtypes of juvenile rheumatoid arthritis. A low frequency of juvenile rheumatoid arthritis has been noted in Oriental children (131,143,145) and an unusually high frequency among British Columbian Indian children (145,146).

There is some evidence of a genetic predisposition to juvenile rheumatoid arthritis (22,23,242) and of a greater than expected number of first-degree relatives of juvenile rheumatoid arthritis cases who have adult rheumatoid arthritis (22,23,186). A subgroup of the pauciarticular onset cases who are HLA B27 positive was mentioned above; reports of associations of juvenile rheumatoid arthritis with other HLA antigens have been inconclusive.

Consideration has been given to the possible role of an infectious agent, given the frequent systemic onset, fever, rash, and enlarged lymph nodes. Initial evidence that the rubella virus might be involved (200,240,241,251) has not been confirmed (17,128,252). No other specific viruses or bacteria have been implicated, despite a variety of serological, immunological, and isolation studies (17,128,150,156,212, 249,252). However, there is still a great deal of interest in the possibility of an infectious etiology. An association between stressful life events and the onset of juvenile rheumatoid arthritis has been suggested (140), but little work in this area has been undertaken.

ANKYLOSING SPONDYLITIS

In ankylosing spondylitis, also called Marie-Strümpell disease, progressive immobility and consolidation of the joints of the spine occurs. Its onset is usually characterized by low back pain, spasm of the paraspinal muscles, and stiffness, especially following periods of inactivity. Often systemic malaise and a raised erythrocyte sedimentation rate are noted. As the disease progresses, changes in the sacroiliac joints may be observed on X-ray, the disease process extends to the thoracic and cervical regions, and in some cases also to the shoulders, hips, knees, and temporomandibular joints. This continuing pathologic process eventually leads to rigidity of the vertebral column with decreased lumbar lordosis, flexed cervical spine, and reduced thoracic, lumbosacral, and hip mobility.

A wide spectrum of severity occurs, ranging from asymptomatic bilateral sacroilitis to severe, deforming, and disabling disease. Polley and Slocumb (253) reported that 72 percent of cases had a prognosis characterized by continuing exacerbations and remissions, while in the remaining 28 percent of cases, the disease pursued a continually disabling course without intermittent remissions. Radford et al. (257) studied the mortality experience of ankylosing spondylitis patients and found increased mortality related to gastrointestinal disease and circulatory diseases, especially in males.

Diagnostic as well as population survey criteria for ankylosing spondylitis were established initially in Rome in 1961 (166) and later modified in New York in 1966 (260). Although these criteria have been criticized as being heavily weighted toward radiographic detection of sacroilitis, they do appear to reflect the general symptomatology of the disease (206). Applying the criteria to females poses special problems, however. Physicians are hesitant to x-ray the sacroiliac area in females of reproductive age; consequently, in population surveys females have been excluded from estimates of prevalence. In addition, because of the well-known male preponderance, radiologists tend not to diagnose definite ankylosing spondylitis in females, even when radiographic evidence of sacrolitis is present (16,18).

Estimates of the prevalence of ankylosing spondylitis differ greatly from one population to another. Much of this variation is believed to be real, despite some differences in the diagnostic criteria used. Recent prevalence estimates in the United States have ranged from 2 to 4 per 1000 in males and from 0.5 to 0.7 per 1000 in females (66,214). In contrast, ankylosing spondylitis has been reported to be virtually absent among aborigines in Australia (73) and extremely rare in black Africans (296). Baum (30) has estimated that American blacks have a prevalence rate one quarter of that in American whites. Among North American Indian tribes, however, prevalence rates have been reported of almost 6 percent in adult male Haida Indians, 1.5 percent among Bella Coolas, and 3.3 percent among Pimas (120,121). Prevalence rates of 4 per 10,000 in Japan (317), 7 per 10,000 in Iraq (13), and 20 per 10,000 in Hungary (123) have been reported.

Evidence from recent studies indicates that prevalence rates of ankylosing spondylitis have generally been underestimated, although there is disagreement about the extent of the underestimation (16,18,63, 71,106,114,207,270). Nevertheless, it is felt that there are indeed large relative differences in prevalence rates, even though the actual values of the prevalence rates may have been underestimated to a certain degree.

There are few reports in the literature examining incidence rates of the disease. However, Carter et al. (66), using data from Rochester, Minnesota, have estimated the annual incidence rate in males to be 1.1 per 10,000 and in females 0.4 per 10,000 over the age range 15 to 74 years.

The age at onset in the vast majority of cases is between 15 and 35 years (159,205,208,253). In less than 10 percent of cases does the onset occur earlier than 15 years, and less than 5 percent of individuals develop symptoms after reaching age 50 years (43,205,277,331).

The ratio of affected males to females is uncertain, although there are considerably more males than females with severe disease. Early reports based on case series seen at selected facilities indicated a male-to-female ratio of about 10 to 1 (253,318,328). However, because the disease is more severe and therefore more easily recognized in males, a higher proportion of males than of females affected with ankylosing spondylitis seeks treatment and is diagnosed (90,155,159,205,207,208,262,318). In females, not only does the disease tend to take a milder course, but there is more peripheral involvement, less frequent ankylosis of the spine, more paravertebral ossification, and more cervical spine involvement, thus making diagnosis more difficult, above and beyond the reluctance of physicians to take X-rays in the pelvic area of females in the age range at highest risk (144,155,159,205,262,318). More recent studies, probably based on a broader spectrum of patients, have indicated that the sex ratio is about 4 to 1 (90,159,205).

Familial aggregation of ankylosing spondylitis has been well recognized (49,77,85,99,142,160,167). Relatives of cases are from 22 to 30 times more likely to develop ankylosing spondylitis than are relatives of individuals in various comparison groups (85,142). However, until the early 1970s no clear-cut mode of inheritance or obvious environmental factor had been identified as a basis for this high degree of familial aggregation.

A major advance in understanding the genetics of ankylosing spondylitis occurred in 1973, when Brewerton et al. (53), Schlosstein et al. (282), and Caffrey and James (61) reported an association between ankylosing spondylitis and the human leukocyte associated (HLA) histocompatibility antigen B27. The HLA system is briefly described on pages 78–79. They found that among Caucasian patients the frequency of the B27 allele ranged from 88 to 96 percent, while this antigen occurred in only 4 to 8 percent of the normal population. These estimates have been confirmed numerous times. Generally, the percentage of Caucasians with ankylosing spondylitis who have HLA-B27 has ranged between 70 and 100 percent while normal population frequencies in Caucasians have ranged from 4 to 10 percent (77,83,90,104,176,220,271,323–325,334). The strong association between HLA-B27 and ankylosing spondylitis has been found to hold for Caucasian females as well as males (144,155,199,273).

Masi and Medgser (207) have noted that much of the geographic variation in prevalence rates of ankylosing spondylitis is associated with varying frequencies of HLA-B27. The frequency of the B27 allele has been shown to be low in black (124,175,176), Japanese (317), and Australian aborigine (73) populations. In contrast, Gofton (120) has found the Haida Indians to have a HLA-B27 frequency as high as 50 percent.

A high prevalence of ankylosing spondylitis and of sacroilitis has been reported in relatives of B27 positive cases (82,148,298,334). More than 50 percent of first-degree relatives of ankylosing spondylitis probands are B27 positive (53) and the prevalence of ankylosing spondylitis is especially high among B27 positive relatives, although moderately elevated prevalence rates may also occur among B27 negative relatives (70,77).

Because 10 to 30 percent of Caucasian ankylosing spondylitis patients are B27 negative, the clinical spectrum of disease has been studied in B27 positive and B27 negative individuals (178,271,325,334). However, no consistent differences in severity have been found. Khan et al. (179) examined disease severity among patients homozygous for B27 and noted that homozygotes exhibit more peripheral joint involvement than heterozygotes. Among B27 negative individuals with ankylosing spondylitis, moderately increased frequencies of HLA-Bw16 and of Cw1 and Cw2 (323,324) and more marked increased frequencies of HLA-Bw22 (relative risk = 16.7) and HLA-Cw1 among females (relative risk = 14.4) (273) have been reported. However, it must be emphasized that sample sizes were fairly small, and these findings remain unconfirmed.

The association between HLA-B27 and ankylosing spondylitis has been explored in other populations, particularly in those with very low and high frequencies of the allele. Sixty-seven percent of ankylosing spondylitis patients among Japanese have been reported to be B27 positive whereas the normal frequency of the allele is close to zero in Japanese (297). In Northern India (287), Iran (84), and the Jewish population of Israel (48) over 90 percent of ankylosing spondylitis patients are B27 positive, while frequencies of this allele in the general population appear to be below 3 percent. Gofton et al. (120) have reported that among Haida Indians, in whom the frequency of the B27 allele approaches 50 percent, nearly 100 percent of ankylosing spondylitis patients are B27 positive. Twenty-five percent of the Bella-Coola Indians are positive for HLA-B27, and nearly 100 percent of afflicted individuals are positive (120). Among Pima Indians, Calin et al. (64) have demonstrated that nearly 50 percent of males with sacroilitis are B27 positive, but only 9 percent of affected females are B27 positive. The association between B27 and ankylosing spondylitis in the American black population is also not as strong as in Caucasians. Most studies (124,175,176,308) have reported that only 40 to 50 percent of black cases are B27 positive. One report (180) indicated that the frequency of the

HLA-B7 allele is significantly elevated among B27 negative black patients.

The well-documented association with HLA-B27 has stimulated searches for relationships between other HLA antigens and ankylosing spondylitis. Several investigators have failed to find associations between HLA-DR antigens and ankylosing spondylitis (47,174,258,268), except for Dejelo et al. (87) who found significantly decreased frequencies of DRw1 and DRw7, and Braun et al. (47) who reported significantly low frequencies of DRw7. Buisseret et al. (56) have observed an excess of the "ZZ" alleles in ankylosing spondylitis patients, although Sjoblom and Wollheim (291) failed to find this difference.

Three general hypotheses have been proposed that could explain the association between the HLA-B27 allele and susceptibility to ankylosing spondylitis. The one that has the most support is that the development of the disease results from a disease-susceptibility gene that is genetically linked to HLA-B27 (70,83,220,248). However, the mode of inheritance of the gene is a subject of disagreement. Percy and Russel (248) have further suggested that the disease susceptibility gene is not in linkage disequilibrium with HLA-B27, but that a defective epistatic interaction exists between the B27 and a disease-susceptibility gene. Individuals possessing both the B27 allele and the disease-susceptibility gene would occur at a low frequency in the population and develop ankylosing spondylitis. Such a mechanism would account for the occurrence of disease in only 5 percent of B27 positive individuals. B27 negative affected individuals in this model would be explained by gene dosage or other factors.

A second hypothesis is that the B27 gene itself is responsible for susceptibility to ankylosing spondylitis (82,334). Brewerton (54) has specified that at least one other gene is necessary for disease susceptibility, although he does not identify it as a "disease susceptibility gene." A third hypothesis, "molecular mimicry," is based on a proposed cross-reaction between viral or bacterial antigens and the HLA-B27 antigen. The antigenic determinants on invading microorganisms would not be recognized as foreign, thus allowing such infectious agents to elude immunological defenses. This would suggest a pathogenetic mechanism for ankylosing spondylitis in which chronic infection leads to the characteristic tissue destruction in the disease (19,94). Circumstantial evidence suggests that the Klebsiella bacterium might be involved in such a process (95,96,116). It has been proposed that because bacterial cell products may have structural and antigenic similarities to the HLA molecule, Klebsiella may indeed be cross-reactive with B27 to produce molecular mimicry (94,96).

Further support for this model comes from knowledge that other reactive arthritides are associated with B27 and occur after bacterial infection, including Reiter's syndrome, Yersinia arthritis, and Salmonella reactive arthritis (94,207).

It is clear that current knowledge cannot adequately explain the associations between HLA-B27 and ankylosing spondylitis. A better understanding must await further research on the nature and regulatory role of the HLA gene products.

GOUT

Gout occurs as a consequence of elevated serum uric acid levels, which in turn result from abnormal purine metabolism. In attacks of gout, urate crystals are deposited in and around the joints of the extremities. In 80 to 90 percent of cases the first attack involves a single joint, and half the time the joint affected is the metatarsophalangeal joint of the big toe (podagra). The insteps, ankles, heels, knees, wrists, fingers, and elbows may also be involved, although usually it is the lower extremities that are affected. Urate deposits (tophi) may sometimes be found in the cartilage of the ear. Acute attacks of gout are of sudden onset, and the involved joints are hot, red, extremely tender, swollen, and inflamed. If not treated, the attack may last from a few hours to several weeks. After the attack has subsided, there are usually no residual joint symptoms. Most patients experience their second attack within three months to two years after their first attack, but in the absence of treatment, the intervals between attacks tend to become shorter over time. If attacks are allowed to continue, they may become polyarticular with systemic symptoms such as fever, malaise, anorexia, and headache (337). Gout may in most instances be successfully treated and prevented with colchicine therapy; when treated with colchicine, most attacks show marked improvement in 24 to 36 hours and can be fully resolved in three to four days (311).

Primary or idiopathic gout occurs because of defects in purine metabolism of unknown origin, while secondary gout results from intake of drugs such as salicylates or diuretics or the presence of another disease such as renal failure, blood dyscrasia, or lead poisoning (183,272, 284,336). It has been estimated (80,272) that about 90 percent of gout is idiopathic. The 10 percent that is secondary will not be considered further here.

On the average, a person is exposed to twenty to thirty years of hyperuricemia before acute gouty arthritis develops. The risk for attacks of gout increases the higher the serum uric acid level. Hyperuricemia results from increased formation or decreased elimination of uric acid. The major sources of overproduction are excess purine biosynthesis, tissue nucleic acid turnover, and purine precursors in the diet. Possible explanations for underexcretion include defects in secretion, poor filtering by the glomerulus of the kidney, and competition for secretory sites in the proximal tubule of the kidney when uric acid would normally be excreted in the urine (183,272).

Gout occurs when urate crystal deposition in the synovium precipitates the inflammatory response, which in turn leads to the characteristic acute arthritis (284). Why the big toe is so frequently involved is curious. Simkin (290) has hypothesized that fluid that has accumulated in the lower extremities during the day is absorbed at night when the legs are elevated. Fluid accumulation during weight bearing may be especially great in the big toe because of degenerative changes resulting from the great amount of stress which the first metatarsophalangeal joint must bear during walking and other activities. When the legs are raised, water evacuates the joint space as much as two times faster than the urate ion does, resulting in transient local elevations in uric acid. If the concentration exceeds the solubility, crystal formation begins, leading to classic podagra. It should be stressed that this is merely a plausible hypothesis, but it is consistent with the observation that symptoms usually start at night (107,337).

Serum Uric Acid in Populations

It is not clear why only certain individuals with hyperuricemia develop clinical gout. Nevertheless, since gout is so closely related to serum uric acid levels, certain aspects of the epidemiology of hyperuricemia will be considered first. The distribution of serum uric acid in most adult populations is bell shaped with a tendency toward positive skewness in both males and females (see Figure 4-3) (134,217,336). Most males have sharp increases in serum uric acid concentrations between 12 and 14 years of age that are related to skeletal and sexual maturation (133). Females tend to show less marked increases in early puberty (133). At ages 15 to 17 years, both males and females have gradually increasing serum uric acid levels, after which levels stabilize. The adult levels are on the average 1.2 mg per 100 ml lower in females than in males (223).

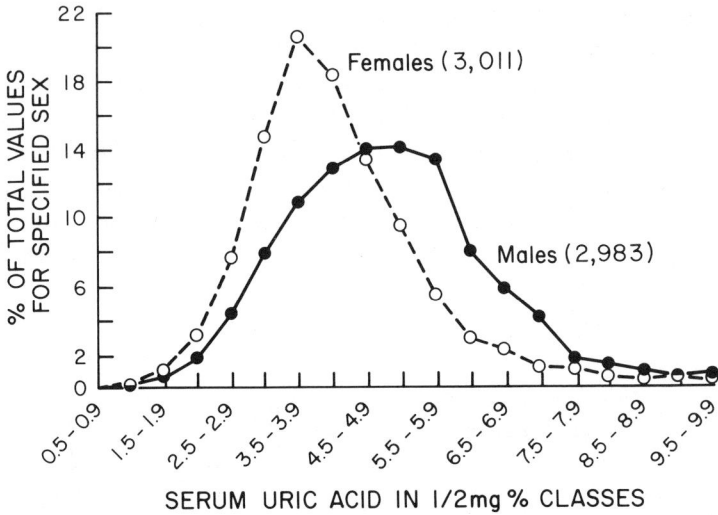

Figure 4-3   Distribution of serum uric acid values. Tecumseh, Mich., 1959–1960. *Source:* Mikkelsen et al. (217).

Around the time of menopause, serum uric acid levels in females gradually increase and approach those of males (127,217,336).

Most populations that have been studied have remarkably similar distributions of serum uric acid levels. Among males, similar distributions have been found in European, Australian, and American Causasians; North American Indians; North American blacks; Japanese; Hawaiians; Chinese; Thais; and Filipinos in the Philippine Islands. In these areas, the mean values of serum uric acid range from 5.0 to 5.7 mg per 100 ml in males (2,27,127,134,153,217,244,254,255,305,319,336). Only isolated surveys, such in Caucasian Australian males (157) and French males (340), have reported somewhat higher mean levels of 6.3 and 5.9, respectively. Female serum uric acid levels have been studied less frequently, but range from 3.7 to 5.0 mg per 100 ml in various Caucasian populations (2,38,127,153,217,244,254,255,305,319,336). Among Japanese in Nagasaki and Hiroshima, mean serum uric acid levels for both males and females were observed to be similar to those for Caucasian populations (163). However, Yano et al. (338) found a somewhat higher mean value, 6.0 mg per 100 ml for Japanese males living in Hawaii. Ethnic groups that exhibit particularly high mean serum uric acid levels are shown in Table 4-5. Surveys in black South Africans and Nigerians have indicated that in urbanized groups both males and females have relatively high

Table 4-5 Ethnic Groups Reported to Have High Mean Serum Uric Acid Levels

American Samoans (134)
Australian aborigines (101)
Chinese in Malaysia (92)
Filipinos in western continental United States and Hawaii (86,137,138,315,336)
Malaysians (58)
Maoris of New Zealand (46,267)
Micronesians of the Western Caroline and Mariana Islands (261,301)
Nauru of the South Pacific (342)
Pukapuka and Rarotonga of the Cook Islands (105)
Xanvante Indians in Brazil (137)

mean uric acid concentrations (35), whereas in rural groups mean values may be lower than those in Caucasian populations (33,112).

Numerous surveys in western Caucasian populations have demonstrated positive associations between serum uric acid and social class (164,182,314,336), although there appear to be some populations where this gradient is not seen (1,27).

While the serum uric acid level generally considered to be hyperuricemic is 7.0 mg per 100 ml or greater in males and 6.0 mg per 100 ml or greater in females (336), these values are somewhat arbitrary and may not be applicable to all populations. The prevalence of hyperuricemia (>7 mg per 100 ml) in males in the Framingham study was 4.8 percent, using a single determination of serum uric acid. However, 9.3 percent of males were hyperuricemic if all determinations over the 14-year period of the study were considered (127). In Tecumseh, Michigan, 6.4 percent of males and 6.3 percent of females were found to be hyperuricemic (>7 mg per 100 ml for males, >6 mg per 100 ml), again using single determinations (217). Prevalence rates of hyperuricemia from other studies show some variability, but in general parallel the trends described above for mean serum uric acid levels. Populations in the South Pacific, for instance, have particularly high prevalence rates of hyperuricemia. The prevalence of hyperuricemia in Maoris exceeds 45 percent in males and 40 percent in females (46,267); a 60 percent prevalence in Naurus was noted (342).

Frequency of Gout and Demographic Chracteristics

Comparison of prevalence rates of gout itself are difficult because of differing diagnostic criteria and methods of study. In general, among pop-

Table 4-6 Percentage of Individuals of Ages 30–59 Who Developed Gout Over a 10-Year Period According to Serum Uric Acid Level on a Single Examination, Framingham, Massachusetts, by Sex

Serum uric acid level (mg/100 ml)	Males		Females	
	Number	Percentage developing gout	Number	Percentage developing gout
<6.0	1615	1.1	2405	0.1
6.0–6.9	354	7.3	71	7.0
7.0–7.9	78	14.2	11	27.2
8.0–8.9	16	18.7	1	—
≥9.0	6	83.3	0	—

Source: Hall et al. (127).

ulations in the United States and Western Europe, prevalence rates of around 0.3 percent have been reported (80,188,337), although rates in France may be higher (340). Male-to-female ratios are about 7 to 1 (80,127,244); prevalence rates are probably highest in the 65 to 74 year age group (244). The age group with the highest incidence rates has varied among the fourth, fifth, and sixth decades in different studies (183).

It was mentioned previously that the risk for gout becomes greater as serum uric acid level increases. In the Framingham study it was found that only 1 percent of males with serum uric acid values below 6.0 mg per 100 ml had gout, in contrast with 83 percent of males with values of 9.0 mg per 100 ml or more (Table 4-6) (127). Accordingly, many of the populations with high mean serum uric acid levels have high prevalence rates of gout. Maori males, for instance, have been reported to have a prevalence rate of 8.8 percent by one group of investigators (46) and 10.2 percent by another (267). High rates are found among South Pacific island groups, including the residents of the Cook Islands (301) and the Micronesian population of Nauru (342), and among Filipino immigrants to the United States (86,315,336). On the other hand, gout has been reported to be rare in blacks (34,139,203,310) and in Australian aborigines (101), despite the relatively high serum uric acid levels of the latter.

In respect to the incidence of gout, annual rates of 1 per 1000 per year have been reported among adults in two Massachusetts communities (127,243). In a recent English survey based on cases seeking medical care, the annual incidence rate was estimated as 3 per 1000 (81). In contrast, Brauer and Prior (46) have reported cumulative eleven-year incidence rates of 10.3 percent in Maori males and 4.3 percent in Maori females.

Suggested Etiologic Agents

Within populations, both hyperuricemia (229,230,239,255,259) and gout (244,255,259,286,341) show familial aggregation, and first-degree relatives of probands with gout have been found to have higher serum uric acid levels than second- or third-degree relatives (229). Although both heredity and environment influence serum uric acid levels, genetic analyses indicate that hyperuricemia is probably influenced more by heredity than environment (113). It is generally agreed that the mode of inheritance of serum uric acid levels is polygenic (42,113,125,229,239,286). However, the mode of inheritance of clinical gout is less clear, and it is likely that environmental factors play a larger role in the etiology of gout itself than in serum uric acid levels.

Although the mechanism of the relationship is not well understood, numerous studies in different populations, races, cultures, and in both sexes have reported strong positive associations between serum uric acid levels and body weight (1,3,33,35,38,39,46,86,105,109,122,127,134,157, 182,233,239,244,254,267,276,299,305,338,341,342). Many surveys have demonstrated that body weight, or closely analogous measures such as surface area and ponderal index, is the single most important correlate of serum uric acid (3,46,109,122,134,157,182,305,338). However, noteworthy exceptions do exist where weight and serum uric acid levels do not appear to be correlated, such as in Australian aborigines (101), Hawaiians (134,136), and Brazilian army recruits (2). Significant correlations have been reported between decreases in plasma uric acid levels and the degree of weight loss in overweight subjects (185,231,285).

Slight positive correlations have also been observed between serum uric acid and intelligence, drive (24), achievement (45), level of professional attainment, leadership, upward striving traits, range of activities, and motivation (24,45,164). Katz and Weiner (164), however, have pointed out that existing evidence does not necessarily support a direct causal link, but rather suggests that associated personality traits are covariates of a third factor. Anxiety, anticipation, and stress have been implicated in temporary changes in serum uric acid levels (161,162,164). In order to estimate the long-term influence of personality traits and emotional status on serum uric acid levels, longitudinally designed studies carefully controlling for hormonal and biochemical variables as well as elements of lifestyle, such as diet, would be necessary (164).

Serum triglycerides, serum cholesterol, blood pressure, alcohol consumption, serum creatinine, glucose levels, diabetes, and coronary atherosclerotic heart disease have been shown to be positively associated with serum uric acid concentrations. Negative associations have been demonstrated for smoking and physical activity. However, different study populations and methods of study have not yielded consistent results, and most of these factors contribute relatively little to explaining variations in serum uric acid levels when compared to the effect of body weight. Furthermore, body weight is independently associated with many of these factors, so that the majority of these variables may be associated with serum uric acid through their underlying correlation with body weight (3,38,39,46,80,100,105,108–110,115,122,134,157,182,222, 233,265,274,314,338,339,341).

"Acculturation" into Westernized society has been shown to raise serum urate levels in Japanese migrants (338), black Africans (33–35), Filipinos (86,315), and New Zealand Maoris (46,267). It has been hypothesized that these increases in serum uric acid levels are related to dietary changes, specifically, increased purine in the diet. Certain ethnic groups may be unable to tolerate increased purine loads in their diet because of genetic susceptibility (267), and Filipinos may have renal defects that induce hyperuricemia when dietary purine levels are increased (135). Klinenberg et al. (184) have proposed that Maoris exhibit abnormally high urate binding, which has a greater relative influence on the development of hyperuricemia than free unbound urate. Hers and Van Den Berghe (141) have suggested that primary hyperuricemia and gout are the result of a single enzyme defect, specifically in the level of adenosine monophosphate deaminase.

Epidemiologic studies do not support a relationship between gout and diabetes mellitus (55,127,213,337,341). Evidence is not consistent regarding an association between gout and hyperlipidemia, hypertension, and atherosclerotic heart disease. To the extent that the associations do exist, these variables are probably related to gout and hyperuricemia through their mutual correlation with obesity (336). Thus, at present, weight is the one known strong correlate of gout, mainly through its association with hyperuricemia.

REFERENCES

1. Acheson, R. M. 1969. "Social class gradients and serum uric acid in males and females." *Brit. Med. J.* 4:65–67.
2. ———. 1970. "Epidemiology of serum uric acid and gout: An example of the complexities of multifactorial causation." *Proc. Roy. Soc. Med.* 63:193–197.
3. ———, and Chan, Y-K. 1969. "New Haven survey of joint diseases. The prediction of serum uric acid in a general population." *J. Chron. Dis.* 21:543–553.

4. ———, Chan, Y.-K., and Clemett, A. R. 1970. "New Haven survey of joint diseases XII: Distribution of symptoms of osteoarthrosis in the hands with reference to handedness." *Ann. Rheum. Dis.* 29:275–286.
5. ———, Chan, Y. K., and Payne, M. 1969. "New Haven survey of joint diseases: The interrelationships between morning stiffness, nocturnal pain and swelling of joints." *J. Chron. Dis.* 21:533–542.
6. ———, and Collart, A. B. 1975. "New Haven survey of joint diseases. XVII. Relationship between some systemic characteristics and osteoarthrosis in a general population." *Ann. Rheum. Dis.* 34:379–387.
7. ———, Kelsey, J. L., and Ginsburg, G. N. 1973. "The New Haven Survey of joint diseases XVI. Impairment, disability, and arthritis." *Brit. J. Prev. Soc. Med.* 27:168–176.
8. Adams, J. C. 1976. *Outline of Orthopaedics.* Edinburgh: Churchill Livingstone.
9. Alder, E., Abramson, J. H., Elkan, Z., Ben Hador, S., and Goldberg, R. 1967. "Rheumatoid arthritis in a Jerusalem population. 1. Epidemiology of the disease." *Amer. J. Epid.* 85:365–377.
10. Allander, E. 1970. "A population survey of rheumatoid arthritis." *Acta. Rheum. Scand. Suppl.* 15, pp. 1–146.
11. ———. 1973. "Conflict between epidemiological and clinical diagnosis of rheumatoid arthritis in a population sample." *Scand. J. Rheum.* 2:109–112.
12. ———. 1976. "Do you die from rheumatism? The five-year mortality in a middle-aged population sample with respect to reported joint symptoms." *Scand. J. Soc. Med.* 4:7–12.
13. Al-Rawi, Z. S., Al-Shakarchi, H. A., Hasan, F., and Thewaini, A. J. 1978. "Ankylosing spondylitis and its association with the histocompatibility antigen HLAB27: An epidemiological clinical study." *Rheumatol. Rehab.* 17:72–75.
14. Alspaugh, M. A., Henle, G., and Henle, W. 1979. "Significance of elevated EBV antibodies in serum or synovial fluids from rheumatoid arthritis patients." *Arth. Rheum.* 22:587.
15. Andersen, S., and Winckler, F. 1979. "The epidemiology of primary osteoarthrosis of the knee in Greenland." *Arch. Orthop. Traumat. Surg.* 93:91–94.
16. Anonymous. 1976. "HLA W27 and ankylosing spondylitis." *Med. J. Aust.* 1:287–288.
17. ———. 1976. "Juvenile rheumatoid arthritis—A viral disease?" *Brit. Med. J.* 2:901–902.
18. ———. 1978. "HLA B27 and risk of ankylosing spondylitis." *Brit. Med. J.* 2:650–651.
19. ———. 1979. "Klebsiella and ankylosing spondylitis—Molecular mimicry?" *Lancet* 1:1012–1013.
20. Ansell, B. M. 1977. "Juvenile chronic polyarthritis." *Arth. Rheum.* 20, Suppl. 2:176–178.
21. ———. 1978. "Chronic arthritis in childhood." *Ann. Rheum. Dis.* 37:107–120.
22. ———, Bywaters, E. G. L., and Lawrence, J. S. 1962. "A family study in Still's disease." *Ann. Rheum. Dis.* 21:243–252.
23. ——— et al. 1969. "Familial aggregation and twin studies in Still's disease, juvenile chronic polyarthritis." *Rheum.* 2:37–61.
24. Anumonye, A., Dobson, J. W., Oppentieim, S., and Sutherland, J. S. 1969. "Plasma uric acid concentrations among Edinburgh business executives." *J. Amer. Med. Ass.* 208:1141–1144.
25. Appleford, D. J. A., and Denman, A. M. 1979. "Fate of Herpes simplex virus in lymphocytes from inflammatory joint effusions II. Mechanisms of non-permissiveness." *Ann. Rheum. Dis.* 38:450–455.

26. Aston, J. N. 1967. *A Short Textbook of Orthopaedics and Traumatology*. Philadelphia: Lippincott.
27. Badley, E. M., Meyrick, J. S., and Wood, P. H. N. 1978. "Gout and serum uric acid levels in the Cotswolds." *Rheum. and Rehab.* 17:133–142.
28. Barada, F. A., O'Brien, W. M., Kay, D., and Horwitz, D. A. 1979. "Defective monocyte cytotoxicity in rheumatoid arthritis." (Proceedings of 43rd Annual Meeting of the ARA.) *Arth. Rheum.* 22:591.
29. Barraclough, D., Russell, A. S., and Percy, J. S. 1977. "Diagnosis and follow-up of children referred to a rheumatic disease unit." *Med. J. Aust.* 1:920–923.
30. Baum, J. 1971. "The rarity of ankylosing spondylitis in the Black race." *Arth. Rheum.* 14:12–18.
31. ———. 1977. "Epidemiology of juvenile rheumatoid arthritis." *Arth. Rheum.* 20, Suppl. 2:158–159.
32. Beasley, R. P., Wilkens, R. F., and Bennett, P. H. 1973. "High prevalence of rheumatoid arthritis in Yakima Indians." *Arth. Rheum.* 16:743–748.
33. Beighton, P., Solomon, L., Soskolone, C. L., and Sweet, B. 1973. "Serum uric acid concentrations in a rural Tswana community in Southern Africa." *Ann. Rheum. Dis.* 32:346–350.
34. ——— et al. 1977. "Rheumatic disorders in the South African Negro. Part IV. Gout and hyperuricemia." *S. Afr. Med. J.* 51:969–972.
35. ———, Solomon, L., Soskolone, C. L., Sweet, B., and Robin, G. 1974. "Serum uric acid concentrations in an urbanized South African Negro population." *Ann. Rheum. Dis.* 33:442–445.
36. ———, Solomon, L., and Valkenburg, H. A. 1975. "Rheumatoid arthritis in a rural South African Negro population." *Ann. Rheum. Dis.* 34:136–141.
37. Bell, D. A., and Block, J. 1979. "Familial rheumatoid arthritis: Clinical, serologic and HLA analysis." (Proceedings of 43rd Annual Meeting of the ARA.) *Arth. Rheum.* 22:592–593.
38. Bengtsson, C., and Tibblin, E. 1977. "Serum uric acid levels in women." *Acta Med. Scand.* 196:93–102.
39. ———, and Tibblin, E. 1977. "On the relationships between age, body weight, serum triglycerides and serum uric acid." (Letter to the editor.) *Acta Med. Scand.* 202:335–336.
40. Bennett, J. C. 1978. "The infectious etiology of rheumatoid arthritis." *Arth. Rheum.* 21:531–537.
41. Bluestone, R., and Pearson, M. 1977. "Ankylosing spondylitis and Reiter's syndrome: Their interrelationship and association with HLA-B27." *Adv. Int. Med.* 22:1–19.
42. Blumberg, B. 1965. "Heredity of gout and hyperuricemia." *Arth. Rheum.* 8:627–647.
43. ———, and Ragan, C. 1956. "The natural history of rheumatoid spondylitis." *Medicine* 35:1–31.
44. Bodmer, M. A. 1978. "The HLA system: Introduction." *Brit. Med. Bull.* 34:213–216.
45. Rose, S., Maheshwari, R., Agarwal, R. C., Bose, S., Dravid, J., and Mathur, R. B. 1977. "Relations of extracurricular activities with serum uric acid, serum cholesterol and fibrinolytic activity in healthy subjects." *J. Assoc. Phys. India* 25:21–23.
46. Brauer, G. W., and Prior, I. A. M. 1978. "A prospective study of gout in New Zealand and Maoris." *Ann Rheum. Dis.* 37:466–472.
47. Braun, W. E., Dejelo, C. L., Clough, J. D., Beck, K. A., Schacter, B. Z., and Khan, M. A. 1978. "No association of known DR antigens with ankylosing spondylitis." *N. Engl. J. Med.* 298:744–745.

48. Brautbar, C., Porat, S., Nelken, D., Gabriel, K. R., and Cohen, T. 1977. "HLA B27 and ankylosing spondylitis in the Israeli population." *J. Rheum.* 4, Suppl. 3:24–32.

49. Bremmer, J. M., Emery, A. E. H., Kellgren, J. H., Lawrence, J. S., and Roth, H. 1968. "A family study in ankylosing spondylitis." In *Population Studies of the Rheumatic Diseases.* P. H. Bennett, and P. H. N. Wood, eds. Amsterdam: Excerpta Medica Foundation, pp. 299–304.

50. ———, Lawrence, J. S., and Miall, W. E. 1968. "Degenerative joint disease in a Jamaican rural population." *Ann. Rheum. Dis.* 27:326–332.

51. Brewer, E. J., Bass, J., Baum, J., Cassidy, J. T., Fink, C., Jacobs, J., Hanson, V., Levinson, J. E., Schaller, J., and Stillman, J. S. 1977. "Current proposed revision of JRA criteria." *Arth. Rheum.* 20:195–198.

52. Brewerton, D. A., Caffrey, M., Nicholls, A., Walters, D., and James, D. C. O. 1973. "Acute anterior uveitis and HL-A27." *Lancet* 2:994–996.

53. ———, Hart, F. D., Nicholls, A., Caffrey, M., James, D. C., and Sturrock, R. D. 1973. "Ankylosing spondylitis and HL-A27." *Lancet* 1:904–907.

54. ———. 1976. "HLA B27 and the inheritance of susceptibility to rheumatic disease." *Arth. Rheum.* 19:656–668.

55. Buchanan, K. D. 1972. "Diabetes mellitus and gout." *Sem. Arth. Rheum.* 2:157–163.

56. Buisseret, P. D., Pembrey, M. E., and Lessof, M. H. 1977. "α_1-anti-trypsin phenotypes in rheumatoid arthritis and ankylosing spondylitis." *Lancet* 2:1358–1359.

57. Bulmash, J. M. 1979. "Rheumatoid arthritis and pregnancy." *Ob. Gyn. Annual* 8:223–276.

58. Burns-Cox, C. J. 1964. "Thirty-three cases of acute arthritis in Sabah." *Med. J. Malaya* 19:25–29.

59. Bywaters, E. G. L. 1968. "Diagnostic criteria for Still's disease (juvenile RA)". In *Population Studies of the Rheumatic Diseases.* P. H. Bennett and P. H. N. Wood, eds. Amsterdam: Excerpta Medica Foundation, pp. 235–240.

60. ———. 1977. "Deaths in juvenile chronic polyarthritis." *Arth. Rheum.* 20, Suppl. 2:256.

61. Caffrey, M., and James, D. C. O. 1973. "Human lymphocyte antigen association in ankylosing spondylitis." *Nature* 242:121.

62. Calabro, J. J., Burnstein, S., and Staley, H. 1977. "JRA posing as a fever of unknown origin." *Arth. Rheum.* 20, Suppl. 2:178–180.

63. Calin, A., and Fries, J. F. 1975. "Striking prevalence of ankylosing spondylitis in "healthy" W27 positive males and females: A controlled study." *N. Engl. J. Med.* 293:835–839.

64. ———, Porta, J., and Fries, J. F. 1977."Clinical history as a screening test for ankylosing spondylitis." *J. Amer. Med. Ass.* 237:2613–2614.

65. Carter, C. O., and Fairbank, T. J. 1974. *The Genetics of Locomotor Disorders.* London: Oxford University Press.

66. Carter, E. T., McKenna, C. H., Brian, D. D., and Kurland, L. T. 1979. "Epidemiology of ankylosing spondylitis in Rochester, Minn. 1935–1973." *Arth. Rheum.* 22:365–370.

67. Cassidy, J. T., and Valkenburg, H. A. 1967. "A 5 year prospective study of rheumatoid factor tests in juvenile rheumatoid arthritis." *Arth. Rheum.* 10:83–90.

68. Cathcart, E. S., and O'Sullivan, J. B. 1970. "Rheumatoid arthritis in a New England town: A prevalence study in Sudbury, Massachusetts." *New Engl. J. Med.* 282:421–424.

69. Cats, A., and Hazevoet, H. M. 1970. "Significance of positive tests for rheumatoid factor in the prognosis of rheumatoid arthritis: A follow-up study." *Ann. Rheum. Dis.* 29:254–260.

70. Christiansen, F. T., Owen, E. T., Dawkins, R. L., and Hanrahan, P. 1977. "Symptoms and signs among relatives of patients with HLA B27 AS: Correlation between back pain, spinal movement, sacroiliitis, and HLA antigens." *J. Rheum.* 4, Suppl. 3:11–17.

71. ———, Hawkins, B. R., Dawkins, R. L., Owen, E. T., and Potter, R. M. 1979. "The prevalence of ankylosing spondylitis among B27 positive normal individuals—A reassessment." *J. Rheum.* 6:713–718.

72. Clarris, B. J. 1978. "Viral arthritis and the possible role of viruses in rheumatoid arthritis." *Aust. N. Z. J. Med.* 8, *Suppl.* 1:40–43.

73. Cleland, L. G., Hay, J. A. R., and Milazzo, S. C. 1975. "Absence of HLA 27 and of ankylosing spondylitis in central Australian aborigines." *Scand. J. Rheum.* 4, Suppl. 8:30.

74. Cobb, S. 1971. *The Frequency of the Rheumatic Diseases.* Cambridge: Harvard University Press.

75. ———, Warren, J. E., Merchant, W. R., and Thompson, D. J. 1957. "An estimate of the prevalence of rheumatoid arthritis." *J. Chron. Dis.* 5:636–643.

76. Cole, B. C., and Cassell, G. H. 1979. "Mycoplasma infections as models of chronic joint inflammation." *Arth. Rheum.* 22:1375–1381.

77. Contu, L., Capelli, P., and Sale, S. 1977. "HLA B27 and ankylosing spondylitis: A population and family study in Sardinia." *J. Rheum.* 4, Suppl. 3:18–23.

78. Crown, S., Crown, J. M., and Fleming A. 1975. "Aspects of the psychology and epidemiology of rheumatoid disease." *Psychol. Med.* 5:291–299.

79. Cunningham, L. 1980. Personal communication.

80. Currie, W. J. C. 1978. "The gout patient in general practice." *Rheum. Rehab.* 17:205–217.

81. ———. 1979. "Prevalence and incidence of the diagnosis of gout in Great Britain." *Ann. Rheum. Dis.* 38:101–106.

82. Daneo, V., Migone, N., Modena, V., Pianchi, S. D., Alfieri, G., Diotallevi, P., Cabonara, A. O., and Piazza, A. 1977. "Family studies and HLA typing in ankylosing spondylitis and sacroilietis." *J. Rheum.* 4, Suppl. 3:5–10.

83. Dausset, J., and Hors, J. 1975. "Some contributions of the HLA complex to the genetics of human diseases." *Transplant. Rev.* 22:44–74.

84. Davatchi, F., Nikbin, B., and Ala, F. 1977. "Histocompatibility antigens in rheumatic diseases in Iran." *J. Rheum.* 4, Suppl. 3:36–38.

85. deBlécourt, J. J., Polman, A., deBlécourt-Meindersma, T. 1961. "Hereditary factors in rheumatoid arthritis and ankylosing spondylitis." *Rheum. Dis.* 20:215–223.

86. Decker, J. L., Healey, L. A., and Skeith, M. D. 1968. "Ethnic variations in serum uric acid: Filipino hyperuricemia, the result of hereditary and environmental factors." In *Population Studies of the Rheumatic Diseases.* P. H. Bennett and P. H. N. Wood, eds. Amsterdam: Excerpta Medica Foundation, pp. 336–343.

87. Dejelo, C. L., Braun, W. E., Khan, M. A., and Clough, J. D. 1978. "HLA-DR antigens and ankylosing spondylitis." *Transplant Proc.* 10:971–972.

88. Denman, A. M. 1978. "Rheumatoid arthritis—A virus disease." *J. Clin. Pathol. Suppl.* 12: 132–143.

89. Depper, J. M., Bardwick, P. A., Bluestein, H. G., Zvaifler, N. J., and Seegmiller, J. E. 1979. "Abnormal regulation of EBV transformation of rheumatoid lymphoid cells." (Proceedings of 43rd Annual Meeting of the ARA.) *Arth. Rheum.* 22:605.

90. Dequeker, J., Decock, T., Walravens, M., and Van De Puttle, I. 1978. "A systematic survey of the HLA B27 prevalence in inflammatory rheumatic diseases." *J. Rheum.* 5:452–459.

91. Dobloug, J. H., Forre, O., and Thorsby, E. 1979. "HLA-DRW4 and rheumatoid arthritis." *Lancet* 1:548–549.

92. Duff, I. F., Mikkelsen, W. M., Dodge, H. J., and Himes, D. S. 1968. "Comparison of uric acid levels in some Oriental and Caucasian groups unselected as to gout or hyperuricemia." *Arth. Rheum.* 11:184–190.

93. Duthie, J. J. R., Brown, P. E., Knox, J. D. E., and Thompson, M. 1957. "Course and prognosis in rheumatoid arthritis." *Ann. Rheum. Dis.* 16:411–424.

94. Ebringer, A. 1979. "Ankylosing spondylitis immune response genes and molecular mimicry." *Lancet* 1:1186.

95. Ebringer, R., Cooke, D., Cawdell, D. R., Cowling, P., and Ebringer, A. 1977. "Ankylosing spondylitis: Klebsiella and HLA B27." *Rheum. Rehab.* 16:190–196.

96. Ebringer, R. W., Cawdell, D. R., Cowling, P., and Ebringer, A. 1978. "Sequential studies in ankylosing spondylitis. Association of Klebsiella pneumonia with active disease." *Ann. Rheum. Dis.* 37:146–151.

97. Edmonds, J., Morris, R. I., Metzger, A. L., Bluestone, R., Terasaki, P. I., Ansell, B., and Bywaters, E. G. L. 1974. "Follow-up study of juvenile chronic polyarthritis with particular reference to histocompatibility antigen w27." *Ann. Rheum. Dis.*, 33:289–292.

98. Edwards, M. H. 1964. "The relationship of the arthritic patient to the community." *J. Amer. Phys. Ther. Ass.* 44:718–723.

99. Emery, A. E. H., and Lawrence, J. S. 1967. "Genetics of ankylosing spondylitis." *J. Med. Genet.* 4:239–244.

100. Emmerson, B. T. 1979. "Atherosclerosis and urate metabolism." *Aust. New Zeal. J. Med.* 9:451–454.

101. ———, Douglas, W., Doherty, R. T., and Feigh, P. 1969. "Serum urate concentrations in the Australian aborigine." *Ann. Rheum. Dis.* 28:150–155.

102. Engel, A. 1968. *Osteoarthritis and Body Measurements.* Publication 1000, No. 29, USPHS, Washington, D.C.

103. Epstein, J. A., Epstein, B. S., Lavine, L. S., Carras, R., Rosenthal, A. D., and Sumner, P. 1973. "Lumbar nerve root compression of the intervertebral foramina caused by arthritis of the posterior facets." *J. Neurosurg.* 39:362–369.

104. Ercilla, M. G., Brancos, M. A., Breysse, Y., Alonso, G., Vives, J., Castillo, R., Rotes Querol, J. 1977. "HLA antigens in Forestier's disease, ankylosing spondylitis, and polyarthrosis of the hands." *J. Rheum.* 4, Suppl. 3:89–93.

105. Evans, J. G., Prior, I. A. M., and Harvey, H. P. B. 1968. "Relation of serum uric acid to body bulk, haemoglobin and alcohol intake in two South Pacific Polynesian populations." *Ann. Rheum. Dis.* 27:319–325.

106. Falace, P., Ruderman, R. J., Ward, F. E., and Swift, M. 1978. "Histocompatibility typing and the counseling of families with ankylosing spondylitis." *Clin. Genet.* 13:380–383.

107. Fessel, W. J. 1978. "Distinguishing gout from other types of arthritis." *Postgrad Med.* 63:134–137.

108. ———. 1980. "High uric acid as an indicator of cardiovascular disease." *Amer. J. Med.* 68:401–404.

109. ———, and Barr, G. D. 1977. "Uric acid, lean body weight, and creatinine interactions: Results from regression analysis of 78 variables." *Sem. Arth. Rheum.* 7:115–121.

110. ———, Siegelaub, A. B., and Johnson, E. S. 1973. "Correlates and consequences of asymptomatic hyperuricemia." *Arch. Int. Med.* 132:44–54.

111. Fink, C. W. 1977. "Patients with JRA: A clinical study." *Arth. Rheum.* 20, Suppl. 2:183–184.

112. Fleischmann, V., and Adadevoh, B. K. 1973. "Hyperuricemia and gout in Nigerians." *Trop. Geogr. Med.* 25:255–261.
113. French, J. G., Dodge, H. J., Kjelsberg, M. O., Mikkelsen, W. M., and Schull, W. J. 1967. "A study of familial aggregation of serum uric acid levels in the population of Tecumseh, Michigan 1959–1960." *Amer. J. Epid.* 86:214–224.
114. Fries, J. F., and Calin, A. 1976. "Ankylosing spondylitis: Genetics vs. environment." *Compr. Ther.* 2:17–22.
115. Garrick, R., Bauer, G. E., Ewan, C. E., and Neale, F. C. 1972. "Serum uric acid in normal and hypertensive Australian subjects." *Austr. New Zeal. J. Med.* 2:351–356.
116. Geczy, A. F., and Yap, J. 1979. "HLAB27, Klebsiella, and ankylosing spondylitis." *Lancet* 1:719–720.
117. Gibofsky, A., Winchester, R. J., Patarroyo, M., Fotino, M., and Kunkel, H. G. 1978. "Disease associations of the Ia-like human alloantigens." *J. Exp. Med.* 148:1728–1732.
118. Gill, D. 1968. "Rheumatic complaints of women using antiovulatory drugs." *J. Chron. Dis.* 21:435–444.
119. Glyn, J. H., Sutherland, I., Walker, G. F., and Young, A. C. 1966. "Low incidence of osteoarthrosis in hip and knee after anterior poliomyelitis: A late review." *Brit. Med. J.* 2:739–742.
120. Gofton, J. P., Chalmers, A., Price, G. E., and Reeve, C. E. 1975. "HLA 27 and ankylosing spondylitis in British Columbia Indians." *J. Rheum.* 2:314–322.
121. ———, Robinson, H. S., and Trueman, G. E. 1966. "Ankylosing spondylitis in a Canadian Indian population." *Ann. Rheum. Dis.* 25:525–527.
122. Goldbourt, U., Medalie, J. H., Herman, J. B., and Neufeld, H. N. 1980. "Serum uric acid: Correlation with biochemical, anthropometric, clinical and behavioral parameters in 10,000 Israeli men." *J. Chron. Dis.* 33:435–443.
123. Gomor, B., Gyodi, E., and Bakos, L. 1977. "Distribution of HLAB27 and ankylosing spondylitis in the Hungarian population." *J. Rheum.* 4, Suppl. 3:33–35.
124. Good, A. E., Kawanishi, H., and Schultz, J. S. 1976. "HLAB27 in Blacks with ankylosing spondylitis or Reiter's disease." *N. Engl. J. Med.* 294:166.
125. Gulbrandsen, C. L., Morton, N. E., Rao, D. C., Rhoads, G. G., and Kagan, A. 1979. "Determinants of plasma uric acid." *Hum. Genet.* 50:307–312.
126. Gunn, D. R. 1974. "Don't sit—squat!" *Clin. Orthop.* 103:104–105.
127. Hall, A. P., Barry, P. E., Dawber, T. R., and McNamara, P. M. 1967. "Epidemiology of gout and hyperurecemia." *Amer. J. Med.* 42:27–37.
128. Hamerman, D. 1975. "Evidence for an infectious etiology of rheumatoid arthritis." *Ann. N.Y. Acad. Sci.* 256:25–38.
129. Hanissian, A. S., Masi, A. T., Kassees-Wahid, L., and Robinson, H. 1977. "Comparison of early patterns of rheumatoid arthritis in juveniles and young adults." *Arth. Rheum.* 20, Suppl. 2:192.
130. Hanson, V., Drexler, E., and Kornreich, H. 1969. "The relationship of rheumatoid factor to age of onset in juvenile rheumatoid arthritis." *Arth. Rheum.* 12:82–86.
131. ———, Kornreich, H., Bernstein, B., King, K. K., and Singsen, B. 1977. "Correlations of age at onset, sex, and serologic factors." *Arth. Rheum.* 20, Suppl. 2:185–186.
132. ——— et al. 1977. "Prognosis of juvenile rheumatoid arthritis." *Arth. Rheum.* 20:279–284.
133. Harlan, W. R., Cornoni-Huntley, J., and Leaverton, P. E. 1979. "Physiologic determinants of serum urate levels in adolescence." *Pediatrics* 63:569–575.

134. Healey, L. A. 1975. "Epidemiology of hyperurecimia." *Arth. Rheum.* 18, Suppl: 709–712.
135. ———, and Bayani-Sioson, P. S. 1971. "A defect in the renal excretion of uric acid in Filipinos." *Arth. Rheum.* 14:721–726.
136. ———, Caner, J. E., Passett, D. R., and Decker, J. L. 1966. "Serum uric acid and obesity in Hawaiians." *J. Amer. Med. Ass.* 196:364–365.
137. ———, and Hall, A. P. 1970. "The epidemiology of hyperuricemia." *Bull. Rheum. Dis.* 20:600–603.
138. ———, Skeith, M. D., Decker, J. L., and Bayani-Sioson, P. S. 1967. "Hyperurecemia in Filipinos: Interaction of heredity and environment." *Amer. J. Hum. Genet.* 19:81–85.
139. Hench, P. S., Bauer, W., Dawson, M. H., Hall, F., Holbrook, W. P., Key, V. A., and McEwen, C. 1940. "The problem of rheumatism and arthritis. Review of American and English literature for 1938." *Ann. Int. Med.* 13:1837–1944.
140. Henoch, M. J., Batson, J. W., and Baum, J. 1978. "Psychosocial factors in juvenile rheumatoid arthritis." *Arth. Rheum.* 21:229–233.
141. Hers, H. G., and Van Den Berghe, G. 1979. "Enzyme defect in primary gout." *Lancet* 1:585–586.
142. Hersh, A. H., Stecher, R. M., Soloman, W. M., Wolpaw, R., and Hauser, H. 1950. "Heredity in ankylosing spondylitis—A study of 50 families." *Amer. J. Hum. Genet.* 2:391–408.
143. Hicks, R. 1977. "Rheumatic diseases in Hawaii." *Arth. Rheum.* 20, Suppl. 2:161.
144. Hill, H. F., Hill, A. G., and Bodmer, J. G. 1976. "Clinical diagnosis of ankylosing spondylitis in women and relation to the presence of HLA B27." *Ann. Rheum. Dis.* 35:267–270.
145. Hill, R. H. 1977. "Juvenile arthritis in various racial groups in British Columbia." *Arth. Rheum.* 20, Suppl. 2:162.
146. ———, and Robinson, H. S. 1969. "Rheumatoid arthritis and ankylosing spondylitis in British Columbia Indians." *Can. Med. Ass. J.* 100:509–511.
147. Hoagkund, F. T., Yau, A.C.M.A, and Wong, W. L. 1973. "Osteoarthritis of the hip and other joints in Southern Chinese in Hong Kong: Incidence and related factors." *J. Bone Jt. Surg. (Amer.)* 55:545–557.
148. Hochberg, M. C., Bias, W. B., and Arnett, F. C. 1978. "Family studies in HLA B27 associated arthritis." *Medicine* 57:463–475.
149. Hoffman, A. L. 1974. "Psychological factors associated with rheumatoid arthritis." *Nursing Res.* 23:218–234.
150. Hoyeraal, H. M., Froland, S. S., and Wisloff, F. 1975. "Lymphocyte populations and cellular immune reactions in juvenile rheumatoid arthritis." *Scand. J. Immun.* 4:801–810.
151. Hutto, J. H., Jr., and Ayoub, E. M. 1977. "Juvenile rheumatoid arthritis." *Arth. Rheum.* 20, Suppl. 2:191.
152. Isomaki, H. A., Mutru, O., and Koota, K. 1975. "Death rate and causes of death in patients with rheumatoid arthritis." *Scand. J. Rheum.* 4:205–208.
153. ———, and Takkunen, H. 1969. "Gout and hyperurecemia in a Finnish rural population." *Acta Rheum. Scand.* 15:112–120.
154. Jaraquemade, D., Pachoula-Papasteriadis, C., Festenstein, H., Sachs, J. A., Roitt, I. M., Corbett, M., and Ansell, B. 1979. "HLA-D and DR determinants in rheumatoid arthritis." *Transpl. Proc.* 11:1306.
155. Jeannet, M., Saudan, Y., and Bitter, T. 1975. "HLA 27 in female patients with ankylosing spondylitis." *Tiss. Ant.* 6:262–264.

156. Jennings, J. 1975. "Defective cellular immunity in juvenile rheumatoid arthritis." *Ann. Rheum. Dis.* 34:196.

157. Jeremy, R., and Towson, J. 1971. "Serum urate levels and gout in Australian males." *Med. J. Aust.* 1:1116–1118.

158. Jonck, L. M. 1961. "The mechanical disturbances resulting from lumbar disc space narrowing." *J. Bone Jt. Surg. (Brit.)* 43:362–375.

159. Julkunen, H. 1962. "Rheumatoid spondylitis." *Acta Rheum. Scand.*, Suppl. 4, 1–110.

160. ———, and Rokkanen, P. 1969. "Ankylosing spondylitis and osteitis condensans ilii." *Acta Rheum. Scand.* 15:224–231.

161. Kasl, S. V., Cobb, S., and Brooks, G. W. 1968. "Changes in serum uric acid and cholesterol levels in men undergoing job loss." *J. Amer. Med. Ass.* 206:1500–1507.

162. ———, and Sandler, D. P. 1977. "An epidemiological study of serum cholesterol and serum uric acid in a population of healthy young men." *Milit. Med.* 142:1:853–857.

163. Kato, H., Duff, I. F., Russell, W. J., Uda, Y., Hamilton, H. B., Kawamoto, S., and Johnson, K. B. 1971. "Rheumatoid arthritis and gout in Hiroshima and Nagasaki." *J. Chron. Dis.* 23:659–679.

164. Katz, J. L., and Weiner, H. 1972. "Psychosomatic considerations in hyperuricemia and gout." *Psychosom. Med.* 34:165–182.

165. Kellgren, J. H. 1954. "Primary generalized osteoarthritis." *Bull. Rheum. Dis.* 4:63–64.

166. ———. 1963. *Symposium on Population Studies in Relation to Chronic Rheumatic Diseases, Rome, 1961.* J. H. Kellgren, M. R. Jeffrey, and J. Ball, eds. Oxford: Blackwell.

167. ———. 1964. "The epidemiology of the rheumatic diseases." *Ann. Rheum. Dis.* 23:109–122.

168. ———, and Lawrence, J. S. 1952. "Rheumatism in miners. Part II. X-ray study." *Brit. J. Ind. Med.* 9:197–207.

169. ———, and Lawrence, J. S. 1956. "Rheumatoid arthritis in a population sample." *Ann. Rheum. Dis.* 15:1–11.

170. ———, and Lawrence, J. S. 1957. "Radiological assessment of osteo-arthrosis." *Ann. Rheum. Dis.* 16:494–501.

171. ———, and Lawrence, J. S. 1958. "Osteo-arthrosis and disk degeneration in an urban population." *Ann. Rheum. Dis.* 17:388–397.

172. ———, Lawrence, J. S., and Beer, F. 1963. "Genetic factors in generalized osteoarthrosis." *Ann. Rheum. Dis.* 22:237–255.

173. ———, and Moore, R. 1952. "Primary generalized osteoarthrosis." *Brit. Med. J.* 1:181–187.

174. Kemple, K., Gatti, R. A., Liebold, W., Klinenberg, J., and Bluestone, R. 1979. "HLA-D locus typing in ankylosing spondylitis and Reiter's Syndrome." *Arth. Rheum.* 22:371–375.

175. Khan, M. A. 1978. "Race related differences in HLA association with ankylosing spondylitis and Reiter's disease in American Blacks and Whites." *J. Nat. Med. Assoc.* 70:41–42.

176. ———, Braun, W. E., Kushner, I., Grecek, D. W., Muir, W. A., and Steinberg, A. G. 1977. "HLA B27 in ankylosing spondylitis: Differences in frequency and relative risk in American Blacks and Caucasians." *J. Rheum.* 4, Suppl. 3:39.

177. ———, Kushner, I., Ballou, S. P., and Braun, W. E. 1979. "Familial rheumatoid arthritis and HLA-DRW4." *Lancet* 921–922.

178. ———, Kushner, I., and Braun, W. E. 1977. "Comparison of clinical features in HLA B27 positive and negative patients with ankylosing spondylitis." *Arth. Rheum.* 20:909–912.

179. ——— et al., 1978. "HLA B27 homozygosity in ankylosing spondylitis: Relationship to risk and severity." *Tiss. Ant.* 11:434–438.

180. ——— et al., 1978. "Subgroup of ankylosing spondylitis associated with HLA B7 in American Blacks." *Arth Rheum.* 21:528–530.

181. King, S. H., and Cobb, S. 1958. "Psychosocial factors in the epidemiology of rheumatoid arthritis." *J. Chron. Dis.* 7:466–475.

182. Klein, R., Klein, B. E., Cornoni, J. C., Maready, J., Cassel, J. C., and Tyroler, H. A. 1973. "Serum uric acid. Its relationship to coronary heart disease risk factors and cardiovascular disease, Evans County, Georgia." *Arch. Intern. Med.* 132:401–410.

183. Klinenberg, J. R. 1977. "Hyperurecemia and gout." *Med. Clin. N. Am.* 61:299–312.

184. ———, Campion, D. S., Olsen, R. W., Caughey, D., and Bluestone, R. 1977. "A relationship between free urate, protein-bound urate, hyperurecemia and gout in Caucasians and Maoris." *Adv. Exp. Med. Biol. (Brit.)* 76:159–162.

185. Krizek, V. 1966. "Serum uric acid in relation to body weight." *Ann. Rheum. Dis.* 25:456–458.

186. Laaksonen, A. L. 1966. "A prognostic study of juvenile rheumatoid arthritis." *Acta Ped. Scand,* Suppl. 166:1–764.

187. Lawrence, J. S. 1955. "Rheumatism in coal miners. Part III Occupational factors." *Brit. J. Ind. Med.* 12:249–261.

188. ———. 1960. "Heritable disorders of connective tissue." *Proc. Roy. Soc. Med.* 52:522–526.

189. ———. 1961. "Prevalence of rheumatoid arthritis." *Ann. Rheum. Dis.* 20:11–17.

190. ———. 1961. "Rheumatism in cotton operatives." *Brit. J. Ind. Med.* 18:270–276.

191. ———. 1969. "The epidemiology and genetics of rheumatoid arthritis." *Rheum. Ann. Report* 2:1–36.

192. ———. 1969. "Generalized osteoarthritis in a population sample." *Amer. J. Epid.* 90:381–389.

193. ———, Bremmer, J. M., Ball, J. A., and Burch, T. A. 1966. "Rheumatoid arthritis in a subtropical population." *Ann. Rheum. Dis.* 25:59–66.

194. ———, Bremmer, J. M., and Bier, F. 1966. "Osteoarthrosis. Prevalence in the population and relationship between symptoms and x-ray changes." *Ann. Rheum. Dis.* 25:1–24.

195. ———, Laine, V. A. I., and deGraff, R. 1961. "The epidemiology of rheumatoid arthritis in Northern Europe." *Proc. Roy. Soc. Med.* 54:454–462.

196. Leach, R. E., Boumgard, S., and Broom, J. 1973. "Obesity: Its relationship to osteoarthritis of the knee." *Clin. Orthop.* 93:271–273.

197. Lee, P., Rooney, P. J., Sturrock, R. D., Kennedy, A. C., and Dick, W. C. 1974. "The etiology and pathogenesis of osteoarthrosis: A review." *Sem. Arth. Rheum.* 3:189–218.

198. Levinson, J. E., Balz, G. P., and Hess, E. V. 1977. "Report of studies on juvenile arthritis." *Arth. Rheum.* 20, Suppl. 2:189–190.

199. Levitin, P. M., Gough, W. W., and Davis, J. S. 1976. "HLA B27 antigen in women with ankylosing spondylitis." *J. Amer. Med. Ass.* 235:2261–2622.

200. Linneman, C. C., Levinson, J. E., Buncher, C. R., and Schiff, G. M. 1975. "Rubella antibody levels in juvenile rheumatoid arthritis." *Ann. Rheum. Dis.* 34:354–357.
201. Linos, A., Worthington, J. W., O'Fallon, W. M., and Kurland, L. T. 1978. "Rheumatoid arthritis and oral contraceptives." *Lancet* 1:871.
202. ———— et al. 1980. "The epidemiology of rheumatoid arthritis: A study of incidence, prevalence and mortality." *Amer. J. Epid.* 111:87–98.
203. Lowenthal, M. N., and Dymond, I. D. 1977. "Gout and hyperurecemia in Blacks."*S. Afr. Med. J.* 52:832.
204. Macnab, I. 1950. "Spondylolisthesis with an intact neural arch—the so-called pseudo-spondylolisthesis." *J. Bone Jt. Surg. (Brit.)* 32:325–333.
205. Masi, A. T. 1978. "HLA B27 and other host interactions in spondyloarthropathy syndromes." *J. Rheum.* 5:359–362.
206. ————, and Medsger, T. A. Jr. 1979. "Epidemiology of the rheumatic diseases." In *Arthritis and Allied Conditions.* D. J. McCarty, ed. Philadelphia: Lea and Febiger, pp. 11–35.
207. ————, and Medsger, T. A. 1979. "New look at the epidemiology of ankylosing spondylitis and related syndromes." *Clin. Orthop.* 143:15–29.
208. McBryde, A. M., Jr., and McCollum, D. E. 1973. "Ankylosing spondylitis in women—The disease and its prognosis." *N. C. Med. J.* 34:34–37.
209. Medsger, A. R., and Robinson, H. 1972. "Comparative study of divorce in rheumatoid arthritis and other rheumatic diseases." *J. Chron. Dis.* 25:269–275.
210. Méndez-Bryan, R., González-Alcover, R., and Roger, L. 1964. "Rheumatoid arthritis: Prevalence in a tropical area." *Arth. Rheum.* 7:171–176.
211. Miall, W. E., Ball, J., and Kellgren, J. H. 1958. "Prevalence of rheumatoid arthritis in urban and rural populations in South Wales." *Ann. Rheum. Dis.* 17:263–272.
212. Middleton, P. J., and Highton, T. C. 1975. "Failure to show mycoplasmas and cytopathogenic virus in rheumatoid arthritis." *Ann. Rheum. Dis.* 34:369–375.
213. Mikkelsen, W. M. 1965. "The possible association of hyperurecemia and/or gout with diabetes mellitus." *Arth. Rheum.* 8:853–864.
214. ————. 1976. "Ankylosing spondylitis." *Arth. Rheum.* 19:1011–1014.
215. ————, and Dodge, H. 1969. "Four year follow-up of suspected rheumatoid arthritis: The Tecumseh, Michigan, Community Health Survey." *Arth. Rheum.* 12:87–91.
216. ————, Dodge, H., Duff, I. F., and Kato, H. 1967. "Estimates of the prevalence of rheumatic diseases in the population of Tecumseh, Michigan 1959–1960." *J. Chron. Dis.* 20:351–359.
217. ————, Dodge, H., and Valkenburg, H. A. 1965. "The distribution of serum uric acid values in a population unselected as to gout or hyperurecemia." *Amer. J. Med.* 39:242–251.
218. ————, Duff, I. F., and Dodge, H. J. 1970. "Age-sex specific prevalence of radiographic abnormalities of the joints of the hands, wrists and cervical spine of adult residents of the Tecumseh, Michigan, community health study area." *J. Chron. Dis.* 23:151–159.
219. Mitchell, G. A. G. 1931. "The significance of lumbosacral transitional vertebrae." *Brit. J. Surg.* 24:147–158.
220. Moller, E., and Olhagen, B. 1975. "Studies on the major histocompatibility system in patients with ankylosing spondylitis." *Tiss. Ant.* 6:237–246.
221. Monson, R. R., and Hall, A. P. 1976. "Mortality among arthritics." *J. Chron. Dis.* 29:459–467.

222. Montoye, H., Mikkelsen, W., Metzner, H., and Keller, J. 1976. "Physical fitness, fatness and serum uric acid." *J. Sports Med. Phys. Fit.* 16:253-260.

223. Munan, L., Kelly, A., and Petitclerc, C. 1977. "Serum urate levels between ages 10 and 14: Changes in sex trends." *J. Lab. Clin. Med.* 90:990-996.

224. Murray, R. O. 1965. "The aetiology of primary osteoarthritis of the hip." *Brit. J. Radiol.* 38:810-824.

225. National Center for Health Statistics. 1966. *Osteoarthritis in Adults by Selected Demographic Characteristics, United States, 1960-1972.* Series 11, No. 20.

226. ————. 1966. *Rheumatoid Arthritis in Adults, United States, 1960-1962.* Series 11, No. 17.

227. ————. 1979. *Basic Data on Arthritis. Knee, Hip, and Sacroiliac Joints, in Adults Ages 25-74 Years, United States, 1971-1975.* Series 11, No. 213.

228. The National Health Education Committee. 1976. *Facts on the Major Diseases in the United States Today.* New York.

229. Neel, J. V. 1968. "The control of blood uric acid levels—A problem in genetic epidemiology." In *Population Studies of the Rheumatic Diseases.* P. H. Bennett and P. H. N. Wood, eds. Amsterdam: Excerpta Medica Foundation, pp. 319-336.

230. ————, Rakic, M. T., Davidson, R. J. Valkenburg, H. A., and Mikkelsen, W. N. 1965. "Studies on hyperurecemia. II. A reconsideration of the distribution of serum uric acid values in the families of Smyth, Cotterman, and Freyberg." *Amer. J. Hum. Genet.* 17:14-22.

231. Nicholls, A., and Scott, J. T. 1972. "Effect of weight-loss on plasma and urinary levels of uric acid." *Lancet* 2:1223-1224.

232. Nijenhuis, L. E. 1977. "Genetic considerations on association between HLA and disease." *Human Genet.* 38:175-182.

233. Noppa, H., Bengtsson, C., Björntorp, P., Smith, U., and Tibblin, E. 1978. "Overweight in women—Metabolic aspects." *Acta Med. Scand.* 203:135-141.

234. Norcross, B. M. 1959. "Juvenile rheumatoid arthritis." *Minn. Med.* 42:1760-1767.

235. Norval, M., and Marmion, B. P. 1976. "Attempts to identify viruses in rheumatoid synovial cells." *Ann Rheum. Dis.* 35:106-113.

236. ————, and Smith, C. 1979. "Search for viral nucleic sequences in rheumatoid cells." *Ann. Rheum. Dis.* 38:456-462.

237. O'Brien, W. M. 1967. "The genetics of rheumatoid arthritis." *Clin. Exp. Immun.* 2:785-802.

238. ————, Bennett, P. H., Burch, T. A., and Bunim, J. J. 1967. "A genetic study of rheumatoid arthritis and rheumatoid factor in Blackfeet and Pima Indians." *Arth. Rheum.* 10:163-179.

239. ————, Burch, T. A., and Bunim, J. J. 1966. "Genetics of hyperuricemia in Blackfeet and Pima Indians." *Ann. Rheum. Dis.* 25:117-119.

240. Ogra, P. L., and Herd, J. K. 1972. "Serologic association of rubella virus infection and juvenile rheumatoid arthritis." *Arth. Rheum.* 15:121.

241. ————, Ogra, S. S., Chiba, Y., and Dzierba, J. L. 1975. "Rubella-virus infection in juvenile rheumatoid arthritis." *Lancet* 1:1157-1161.

242. Omenn, G. S. 1977. "Genetics of rheumatic diseases." *Arth. Rheum.* 20, Suppl. 2:473-483.

243. O'Sullivan, J. B. 1968. "The incidence of gout and related uric acid levels in Sudbury, Mass." In *Population Studies of the Rheumatic Diseases.* P. H. Bennett and P. H. N. Wood, eds. Amsterdam: Excerpta Medica Foundation, pp. 371-375.

244. ———. 1972. "Gout in a New England town: A prevalence study in Sudbury, Mass." *Ann. Rheum. Dis.* 31:166–169.

245. Paget, S. A., and Gibofsky, A. 1979. "Immunopathogenesis of rheumatoid arthritis." *Amer. J. Med.* 67:961–970.

246. Panayi, G. S., Wooley, P. H., and Batchelor, J. 1978. "Genetic basis of rheumatoid disease: HLA antigens, disease manifestations, and toxic reactions to drugs." *Brit. Med. J.* 2:1326–1328.

247. Partridge, R. E. H., and Duthie, J. J. R. 1968. "Rheumatism in dockers and civil servants: A comparison of heavy manual and sedentary workers." *Ann. Rheum. Dis.* 27:559–568.

248. Percy, J. S., and Russel, A. S. 1975. "Prevalence of ankylosing spondylitis and its association with HL-A27." *J. Rheum.* 2:351–354.

249. Person, D. A., and Sharp, J. T. 1976. "The etiology of rheumatoid arthritis." *Bull. Rheum. Dis.* 27:888–891.

250. Phillips, P. E. 1971. "Virologic studies in rheumatoid arthritis and other connective tissue diseases." *J. Exp. Med.* 134:3135–3195.

251. ———. 1973. "Viral antibody and IgG levels in juvenile rheumatoid arthritis." *Arth. Rheum.* 16:126.

252. ———. 1977. "The role of infectious agents in childhood rheumatic diseases." *Arth. Rheum.* 20, Suppl. 2:459–466.

253. Polley, H. F., and Slocumb, C. H. 1949. "Rheumatoid spondylitis: A study of 1035 cases." *Ann. Int. Med.* 26:240–249.

254. PongPaew, P., Saovakontha, S., and Schelp, F. P. 1977. "Serum uric acid level of Thai individuals in comparison with the nutritional status and some other physical and biochemical parameters." *Amer. J. Clin. Nutr.* 30:2122–2125.

255. Popert, A. J., and Hewitt, J. V. 1962. "Gout and hyperurecemia in rural and urban populations." *Ann. Rheum. Dis.* 21:154–162.

256. Puranen, J., Ala-Ketola, L., Peltokallio, P., and Saarela, J. 1975. "Running and primary osteoarthritis of the hip." *Brit. Med. J.* 2:424–425.

257. Radford, E. P., Doll, R., and Smith, P. G. 1977. "Mortality among patients with ankylosing spondylitis not given x-ray therapy." *N. Engl. J. Med.* 297:572–582.

258. Raffoux, C., Faure, G., Netter, P., Streiff, R., Pourel, J., and Gaucher, A. 1978. "No association of DRW antigens with ankylosing spondylitis." *Arth. Rheum.* 21:997.

259. Rakic, M. T., Valkenburg, H. A., Davidson, R. T., Engels, J. P., Mikkelsen, W. M., Neel, J. V., and Duff, I. F. 1964. "Observations on the natural history of hyperurecemia and gout." *Amer. J. Med.* 37:862–871.

260. "Recommendations." 1968. In *Population Studies of the Rheumatic Diseases.* P. H. Bennett and P. H. N. Wood, eds. Amsterdam: Excerpta Medica Foundation, pp. 457–458.

261. Reed, D., Labarthe, D., and Stallones, R. 1972. "Epidemiologic studies of serum uric acid levels among Micronesians." *Arth. Rheum.* 15:381–390.

262. Resnick, D., Dwosh, I. L., Goergen, T. G., Shapiro, R. F., Utsinger, P. D., Wiesner, K. B., and Bryan, B. L. 1976. "Clinical and radiographic abnormalities in ankylosing spondylitis: A comparison of men and women." *Radiology* 119:293–297.

263. Rimon, R. 1969. "A psychosomatic approach to rheumatoid arthritis." *Acta Rheum. Scand.* Suppl. 13:1–154.

264. Roitt, I. 1977. *Essential Immunology.* Oxford: Blackwell.

265. Rondier, J., Truffert, J., le Go, A., Cayla, J., Hila, A., deGennes, J. L., and Dellebarre, F. 1977. "Gout and hyperlipidaemia—Effect of overweight on the levels of circulating lipids." *Ann. Clin. Res.* 9:239–245.

266. Ropes, M. W., Bennett, G. A., Cobb, S., Jacox, R., and Jessar, R. A. 1958. "Revision of diagnostic criteria for rheumatoid arthritis." *Bull. Rheum. Dis.* 9:175–176.

267. Rose, B. S. 1975. "Gout in the Maoris." *Sem. Arth. Rheum.* 5:121–245.

268. Roy, R., Hébert, J., Latulippe, L., and Latulippe, L. 1979. "Possible association between HLA-D locus and ankylosing spondylitis." *Arth. Rhem.* 22:94–95.

269. Ruderman, R. J., and Ward, F. E. 1977. "HLA B27 in Black patients with ankylosing spondylitis." *Lancet* 1:610.

270. Russell, A. S. 1979. "The prevalence of ankylosing spondylitis." *J. Rheum.* 6:603–605.

271. ———, Lentle, B. C., and Schlaut, J. 1976. "Radiologic and Scintiscan findings in HLA B27 negative patients with ankylosing spondylitis." *J. Rheum.* 3:321–323.

272. Ryckewaert, A., and Kuntz, D. 1974. "Etiologic varieties of hyperurecemia and gout." *Adv. Nephrol.* 3:29–49.

273. Säfwenberg, J., Domeij-Nyberg, and Kjallman, M. 1978. "HLA antigens in females with ankylosing spondylitis and other forms of seronegative rheumatic diseases." *Scand. J. Rheum.* 7:177–182.

274. Saker, P. M., Tofler, O. B., Burvill, M. J., and Reilly, K. A. 1967. "Alcohol consumption and gout." *Med. J. Austr.* 1:1213–1216.

275. Saville, P. D., and Dickson, J. 1968. "Age and weight in osteoarthritis of the hip." *Arth. Rheum.* 11:635–644.

276. Schaffalitzky de Muckadell, O. B., and Gyntelberg, F. 1976. "Occurrence of gout in Copenhagen males, aged 40–59." *Int. J. Epid.* 5:153–158.

277. Schaller, J. G. 1976. "Ankylosing spondylitis of childhood onset." *Arth. Rheum.* 20:398–401.

278. ———. 1977. "Juvenile rheumatoid arthritis." *Postgrad. Med.* 61:177–184.

279. ———. 1977. "Juvenile rheumatoid arthritis." *Arth. Rheum.* 20, Suppl. 2:165–170.

280. ———, and Wedgwood, R. J. 1972. "Juvenile rheumatoid arthritis: A review." *Pediatrics* 50:940–953.

281. Schlesinger, B. E., Forsyth, C. C., White, R. H. R., Smellie, J. M., and Stroud, C. E. 1961. "Observations on the clinical course and treatment of one hundred cases of Still's disease." *Arch. Dis. Child.* 36:65–76.

282. Schlosstein, L., Terasaki, P. I., Bluestone, R., and Pearson, C. M. 1973. "High association of an HLA antigen, W27 with ankylosing spondylitis." *N. Engl. J. Med.* 288:704–706.

283. Schmid, F. R. 1978. "A current definition of rheumatoid arthritis." *J. Chron. Dis.* 31:371–373.

284. Scott, J. T. 1978. "New knowledge of the pathogenesis of gout." *J. Clin. Pathol.* Suppl. 12:205–213.

285. ———, and Sturge, R. A. 1977. "The effect of weight loss on plasma and urinary uric acid and lipid levels." *Adv. Exp. Bio. (Brit.)* 76:274–277.

286. Seegmiller, J. E. 1975. "Genetic considerations of gout." *Arth. Rheum.* 18, Suppl:743–746.

287. Sengupta, S., Sehgal, S., Aikat, B. K., Deodhar, S. D., and James, D. C. O. 1977. "HLAB27 in ankylosing spondylitis in India." *Lancet* 1:1209–1210.

288. Shichikawa, K., Mayeda, A., Komatsubara, Y., Yamamoto, T., Akabori, O., Hongo, I., Kosugi, T., Miyauchi, T., Orihara, M., and Taniguchi, A. 1966. "Rheumatic complaints in urban and rural populations in Osaka." *Ann. Rheum. Dis.* 25:25–31.

289. Silberberg, M., Janett, S. F., and Silberberg, R. 1956. "Obesity and degenerative joint disease." *Arch. Pathol.* 61:280–288.

290. Simkin, P. A. 1977. "The pathogenesis of podagra." *Ann. Int. Med.* 86:230–233.
291. Sjoblom, K. G., and Wollheim, F. A. 1977. "Alpha-1 antitrypsin phenotypes and rheumatic disease." *Lancet* 2:41–42.
292. Slaughter, L., Carson, D. A., Jensen, F. C., Holbrook, T. L., and Vaughan, J. M. 1978. "In vitro effects of Epstein-Barr virus on peripheral blood mononuclear cells from patients with rheumatoid arthritis and normal subjects." *J. Exp. Med.* 148:1429–1434.
293. Smith, C. A. 1979. "On a possible viral eitology of rheumatoid arthritis (Editorial)." *J. Rheum.* 6:113–116.
294. Sokoloff, L., Mickelson, O., Silverstein, E., Jay, G. E., Jr., and Yamamoto, R. S. 1960. "Experimental obesity and osteo-arthrosis." *Amer. J. Phsyiol.* 198:765–770.
295. Solomon, L., Beighton, P., and Lawrence, J. S. 1975. "Rheumatic disorders in the South African Negro. Part II. Osteoarthrosis." *S. Afr. Med. J.* 1737–1740.
296. ———, Beighton, P., Valkenburg, H. A., Robin, G., and Soskolne, C. L. 1975. "Rheumatic disorders in the South African Negro. Part I. Rheumatoid arthritis and ankylosing spondylitis." *South Afr. Med. J.* 49:1292–1296.
297. Sonozaki, H., Seki, H., Chang, S., Machiko, O., and Takeo, J. 1975. "Human lymphocyte antigen, HLA 27 in Japanese patients wtih ankylosing spondylitis." *Tiss. Ant.* 5:131–136.
298. Spencer, D. G., Dick, H. M., Ferguson-Smith, M. A., El-Ghobarey, A. F., and Dick, W. C. 1978. "Genotypic and phenotypic family studies of individuals homozygous and heterozygous for HLAB27, with and without ankylosing spondylitis." *Scott. Med. J.* 23:312–313.
299. Stanhope, J. M., and Prior, I. A. M. 1975. "Uric acid, joint morbidity, and streptococcal antibodies in Maori and European teenagers." *Ann. Rheum. Dis.* 34:359–363.
300. Stastny, P. 1978. "Association of the B-cell alloantigen DRW4 with rheumatoid arthritis." *New Engl. J. Med.* 298:869–871.
301. Steuermann, N., and Farias, A. H. 1960. "Hyperuricemia in Filipinos." *Hawaii Med. J.* 20:151–153.
302. Stewart, S. M., and McBridge, W. H. 1975. "Mycoplasmas and diptheroids in rheumatoid arthritis." *Rheum. Ann. Rev.* 6:329–337.
303. Stillman, J. S., and Barry, P. E. 1977. "Juvenile rheumatoid arthritis." *Arth. Rheum.* 20, Suppl. 2:171–175.
304. Strecher, R. M. 1948. "Heberden's nodes: The clinical characteristic of osteoarthritis of the fingers." *Ann. Rheum. Dis.* 7:1–8.
305. Sturge, R. A., Scott, J. T., Kennedy, A. C., Hart, D. P., and Buchanan, W. W. 1977. "Serum uric acid in England and Scotland." *Ann. Rheum. Dis.* 36:420–427.
306. Sullivan, D. B., Cassidy, J. T., and Petty, R. E. 1975. "Pathogenic implications of age of onset in juvenile rheumatoid arthritis." *Arth. Rheum.* 18:251–255.
307. Svartz, N. 1975. "The origin of rheumatoid arthritis." *Rheum. Ann. Rev.* 6:322–328.
308. Swezey, R., Zucker, L., and Terasaki, P. 1974. "Reduced prevalence of HLA antigen W27 in Black females with ankylosing spondylitis." *J. Rheum.* 1, Suppl. 1:15.
309. Symposium on the Epidemiology of Chronic Rheumatism. 1963. Volume II. *Atlas of Standard Radiographs of Arthritis.* Oxford: Blackwell.
310. Talbott, J. H., Gottlieb, N., Grendelmeier, P., and Rodriquez, E. 1975. "Gouty arthritis in the Black race." *Sem. Arth. Rheum.* 4:209–240.

311. ———, and Yü, T-F. 1976. *Gout and Uric Acid Metabolism*. New York: Stratton Intercontinental Medical Book Corporation.
312. Tan, E. M., Jensen, F. C., Alspaugh, M. A., and Rabin, H. 1979. "Infection with EB virus and rheumatoid arthritis." *Lancet* 1:549.
313. Thomsen, M., Morling, N., Shorrason, E., Svejgaard, A., and Sorenson, S. F. 1979. "HLA-DW4 and rheumatoid arthritis." *Tiss. Ant.* 12:56–60.
314. Thorpe, J. J., and Daley, J. M. 1971. "Hyperuricemia and gout in an employee population." *J. Occup. Med.* 13:524–534.
315. Torralba, T. P., and Bayani-Sioson, P. S. 1975. "The Filipino and gout." *Sem. Arth. Rheum.* 4:307–320.
316. Toyoda, K., Saito, S., Konomi, K., Yamamoto, H., Nobunaga, M., Nomoto, K., and Takeya, K. 1977. "HLA antigens in classical and malignant rheumatoid arthritis in Japanese population." *Tiss. Ant.* 10:56–59.
317. Tsujimoto, M. 1978. "Epidemiologic research on the prevalence of ankylosing spondylitis." *Med. J. Osaka Univ.* 28:363–381.
318. Tyson, T. L., Thompson, W. A. L., and Ragan, C. 1953. "Marie Strümpell spondylitis in women." *Ann. Rheum. Dis.* 12:40–42.
319. Tzonchev, V. T., Shubarov, K., and Illinov, P. 1968. "Prevalence of gout and hyperuricemia in Bulgaria." In *Population Studies of the Rheumatic Studies*. P. H. Bennett and P. H. N. Wood, eds. Amsterdam: Excerpta Medica Foundation, pp. 363–364.
320. Udin, J., Kraus., A. S., and Kelly, H. G. 1970. "Survivorship and death in rheumatoid arthritis." *Arth. Rheum.* 13:125–130.
321. Valkenburg, H. A. 1963. "Rheumatoid factor in populations." In *Epidemiology of Chronic Rheumatism*. Vol. 1. J. H. Kellgren, M. R. Jeffrey, and J. Ball, eds. Philadelphia: Davis, pp. 74–81.
322. ———, Hijmans, W., and Klein, F. 1968. "Rheumatoid factor in patients suffering from chronic infectious diseases living in various temperate and non-temperate areas." In *Population Studies of the Rheumatic Diseases*. P. H. Bennett and P. H. N. Wood, eds. Amsterdam: Excerpta Medica Foundation, pp. 181–191.
323. Van den Berg-Loonen, E. M., Dekker- Saeys, B. J., Meuwissen, S. G. M., and Nijenhuis, L. E. 1977. "Histocompatibility antigens and other markers in ankylosing spondylitis and inflammatory bowel diseases." *J. Rheum.* 3, 4, Suppl. 3:57–59.
324. ———, E. M., Dekker-Saeys, B. J., Meuwissen, S. G. M. and Engelfriet, C. J. 1977. "Histocompatibility antigens and other genetic markers in ankylosing spondylitis and inflammatory bowel diseases." *J. Immunogenet.* 4:167–175.
325. Van der Linden, J. M. J. P., de Ceulaer, K., Van Romunde, L. K. J., and Cats, A. 1977. "Ankylosing spondylitis without HLA B27." *J. Rheum.* 4, Suppl. 3:54–56.
326. Vaughan, J. H. 1979. "Rheumatoid arthritis, rheumatoid factor and the Epstein-Barr virus." *J. Rheum.* 6:381–388.
327. Weiner, H. 1977. *Psychobiology and Human Disease*. New York: Elsevier.
328. West, H. F. 1949. "The aetiology of ankylosing spondylitis." *Ann. Rheum. Dis.* 8:143–149.
329. Wilkes, E., and Meek, E. S. 1979. "Rheumatoid arthritis: Review of searches for an infectious cause I." *Infection* 7:125–128.
330. ———, and Meek, E. S. 1979. "Rheumatoid arthritis: Review of searches for an infectious cause II." *Infection* 7:192–197.

331. Wilkinson, M., Bywaters, E. G. L. 1958. "Clinical features and course of ankylosing spondylitis as seen in a follow-up of 222 hospital referred cases." *Ann. Rheum. Dis.* 17:209–228.
332. Wingrave, S. J., and Kay, C. R. 1978. "Reduction in incidence of rheumatoid arthritis associated with oral contraception." *Lancet* 1:569–571.
333. Wood, P. H. N. 1970. "Epidemiology of rheumatic disorders." *Proc. Roy. Soc. Med.* 63:189–193.
334. Woodrow, J. C., and Eastmond, C. J. 1978. "HLA B27 and the genetics of ankylosing spondylitis." *Ann. Rheum. Dis.* 37:504–509.
335. Wright, E. C., and Acheson, R. M. 1970. "New Haven Survey of Joint Diseases. XI. Observer variability in the assessment of x-rays for osteoarthrosis of the hands." *Amer. J. Epid.* 91:378–392.
336. Wyngaarden, J. B., and Kelley, W. N. 1976. *Gout and Hyperurecemia.* New York: Grune and Stratton.
337. ———, and Kelley, W. N. 1978. "Gout." In *The Metabolic Basis of Inherited Disease.* J. B. Stanbury, J. B. Wyngaarden, and D. S. Fredrickson, eds. New York: McGraw-Hill, pp. 916–1010.
338. Yano, K., Rhoads, G. G., and Kagan, A. 1977. "Epidemiology of serum uric acid among 8000 Japanese-American men in Hawaii." *J. Chron. Dis.* 30:171–184.
339. Yu, T-F. 1977. "Some unusual features of gouty arthritis in females." *Sem. Arth. Rheum.* 6:247–255.
340. Zalokar, J., Lellouch, J., Claude, J. R., and Kuntz, D. 1972. "Serum uric acid in 23,923 men and gout in a subsample of 4257 men in France." *J. Chron. Dis.* 25:305–312.
341. ——— et al. 1974. "Epidemiology of serum uric acid and gout in Frenchmen." *J. Chron. Dis.* 27:59–75.
342. Zimmet, P. Z., Whitehouse, S., Jackson, I., and Thomas, K. 1978. "High prevalence of hyperurecemia and gout in an urbanized Micronesian population." *Brit. Med. J.* 1:1237–1239.

5 Osteoporosis, Osteomalacia and Rickets, and Paget's Disease of Bone

Osteoporosis, osteomalacia, and rickets affect several bones throughout the body and are frequently classified under the heading of Generalized Diseases of the Bone. Paget's disease also often involves more than one bone, but it is perhaps best described as multifocal rather than generalized. Osteoporosis is very common among the elderly of Western countries. Its epidemiology has been studied to a greater extent than that of many other diseases of the musculoskeletal system and several risk factors have been identified. In many of these studies hip fracture has been used as an indicator of the presence of osteoporosis. Osteomalacia and rickets, on the other hand, are uncommon in most Western countries, but are frequently seen in other areas of the world. The major etiologic determinants of osteomalacia and rickets are well established. Paget's disease of bone, although found at autopsy in 3 to 4 percent of adults in Western countries and although of known importance as a risk factor for bone neoplasms in the elderly, has been the subject of little epidemiologic study.

OSTEOPOROSIS

Osteoporosis is a condition in which the density of bone is diminished. Although bone remains biochemically normal, there is reduced bone mass per unit volume of anatomical bone. The disease process occurs in both the bone matrix and calcium, and affects trabecular (spongy) bone to a greater extent than cortical (compact) bone. Depending on the extent of bone loss, osteoporosis may be symptomless or it may be associated with pain, especially in the lower back as a result of compression fractures of lumbar or thoracic vertebrae. Height loss, an increase in abdominal skin folds, and a rounded appearance in the dorsal region of the spine (dowager's hump) may also occur as the disease progresses. The decreased bone density greatly increases the likelihood of fractures; osteoporosis is the most important underlying cause of fractures in the elderly, especially fractures of the vertebrae, hips, and lower arms. In fact, it has been estimated that 70 percent of fractures sustained by women 45 years of age and older in the United States are related to osteoporosis (77).

There is no general agreement about diagnostic criteria for osteoporosis. Frequently used methods of measuring the condition include X-ray measurement of cortical width in long bones, radiodensitometry measurement by comparison with standards, and photon-beam absorptiometry. These methods are subject to various technical difficulties and, in addition, the findings in one bone may not be indicative of the extent of osteoporosis in other bones. Perhaps of greater importance is the question of whether osteoporosis is a normal part of aging or whether it is a disease process. It has been argued (109) that patients said to have osteoporosis are selected from one end of a continuous distribution. Nevertheless, since osteoporosis predisposes to fractures, which are in turn associated with significant morbidity and mortality, it seems reasonable to regard osteoporosis as a disease process (112). Because of the difficulties in diagnosis and definition, much information on the epidemiology of osteoporosis is based on surrogate indicators of osteoporosis such as hip fractures, although some epidemiologic studies have been based on X-ray evidence of decreased bone density in the spine or in other bones.

Osteoporosis may be idiopathic or secondary to conditions such as hormonal defects, nutritional defects, connective tissue disorders of bone marrow, or certain drug therapies. Since the vast majority of cases are idiopathic, this discussion will be limited to epidemiologic characteristics of idiopathic osteoporosis.

Frequency and Demographic Characteristics

The two most marked epidemiologic features of idiopathic osteoporosis are that women are much more frequently affected than men, and that the prevalence increases steeply with age. Starting at about the age of 40, bone mass starts to decrease in both men and women and in both blacks and whites, but the most rapid decrease occurs in white women. These decreases tend to continue throughout the lifespan (10,18,57,99,112,113), although the rate of loss may vary from one individual to another, and may even reverse itself in some individuals for a period of time (73). Eventually, women may lose about one-half and men almost one-quarter of the trabecular bone they had in early adulthood (10).

Table 5-1 shows prevalence rates of osteoporosis, as indicated from X-rays of the lumbar spine, in Michigan women 45 years of age and older; in this study, attempts were made to exclude cases of secondary osteoporosis. It may be seen that more than half of women of age 45 years and older have radiographic evidence of osteoporosis in their lumbar spines (77). Above the age of 75 years, the prevalence is almost 90 percent. In several studies it has been found that fractures associated with osteoporosis occur much more frequently in women than in men and occur more often with increasing age (12,22,27,31,83,87,88,94,168).

Various types of evidence show that osteoporosis is more common among whites than blacks. In both skeletons (158) and living beings (34) the density of bones of blacks is greater than that in whites, and the age-associated decreases in the cortical thickness of bones are greater in whites than blacks (150). Fractures associated with osteoporosis occur less frequently in black populations than in whites, even when age is taken into account (25,46,76,111,152). Hip fractures have been found to be rare in black populations throughout Africa (111).

It might also be noted that hip fracture incidence rates are low among

Table 5-1 Prevalence Rates* of Osteoporosis in Michigan Women of Age 45 and Older, by Age Group

Age group (in years)	Number of women	Percentage with osteoporosis
45–49	290	17.9
50–54	309	39.2
55–59	514	57.7
60–64	426	65.5
65–69	299	73.5
70–74	177	84.2
≥75	73	89.0
Total	2088	56.7

*Prevalence rates are based on X-rays of the lumbar spine.

Source: A. P., Iskrant and R. Smith, Jr. (77).

Asian and African women living in Jerusalem (88) and among Maori women in New Zealand (145). However, in geographic areas where overall incidence rates for hip fractures are low, rates at older ages are similar in the two sexes or are even higher for males than females (145,152–155,168).

Suggested Etiologic Agents

The rapid rate of bone loss in middle-aged and older women has long been thought to be related to the absence or decreased production of ovarian hormones (9). Considerable attention has thus been focused on the role of estrogens. Although it has been established that estrogens cannot restore bone already lost (10,135,136,151), estrogen replacement therapy does appear to decrease the amount of bone that would otherwise be lost, at least as long as the estrogen is being taken. Studies of oophorectomized women have shown that estrogen replacement therapy inhibits bone resorption and thus preserves bone mass. The length of time estrogen replacement therapy has been used is positively associated with thickness of bone, and the shorter the delay between oophorectomy and estrogen use, the less the bone loss (5,6,98,100,159). Withdrawal of estrogen from these women has resulted in the loss of bone mineral content at a rate similar to that in oophorectomized women not given estrogen replacement therapy (89). This finding provides further evidence of an etiologic role for estrogen, but also implies that short-term use of estrogen merely delays the osteoporotic process. Studies in women with intact ovaries have also shown that exogenous estrogens will prevent or arrest bone loss (38,39,67,90,96,108,135). Furthermore, the risk for fractures of the hip and forearm in postmenopausal women is reduced by about 50 percent among women who have used estrogen replacement therapy, although this protective effect appears to be limited to current or recent users (75,79,85,115,165). The reduction in risk is most marked for women who have been using the compounds for five years or more (75,165) and does not seem to depend to any great extent on the dose of estrogen used (165). One study (62) suggests that steroid contraceptives may enhance bone mineralization in some young women.

The relationship of other reproductive variables, including parity, previous breast feeding, and age at menopause to osteoporosis or to hip fractures has not been established (11,56,62,82,85,94).

Thinness (low weight relative to height) has been found to be associated with hip fracture (11,75,85,94) and vertebral crush fractures (143).

Possible underlying mechanisms for this association are (1) greater peripheral estrogen production in obese postmenopausal women (63,90), (2) greater effect of bone loss in women who have less bone mass to begin with, and (3) an ability of heavier people to withstand falls better because of the greater amount of natural padding in their hips, in which case thinness would not be considered a risk factor for osteoporosis but rather for fractures. However, the finding of a positive association between thinness and vertebral crush fractures suggests that lack of natural padding is not the only explanation.

Dietary elements such as calcium, fluoride, and vitamin D are considered by many to be involved in the etiology of osteoporosis, but critical examination of the evidence indicates that little is known with certainty in humans. Animals who have been fed low-calcium diets tend to develop osteoporosis through hyperparathyroidism (80); an increase in parathyroid hormone results in a decrease in calcium content of bone with subsequent increase in serum calcium levels. It therefore seems reasonable that a low-calcium diet would contribute to bone loss in humans once the level of calcium excreted is greater than the amount of calcium absorbed. Among the cross-cultural studies that support a role for calcium, it has been noted that the Finns, who have a high-calcium intake, have low prevalence rates of osteoporosis (111), and that calcium consumption is higher in Puerto Rican and black American women than in white American women, a finding consistent with measures of vertebral atrophy among women in these groups (150). On the other hand, international comparisons among Bantu, Chinese, and Western European populations indicate that dietary calcium is not an important determinant of osteoporosis prevalence (31). There is apparently no evidence that people in developing countries with low-calcium intake have particularly high rates of osteoporosis (117,164). In these comparisons of different population groups many other differences are of course present besides calcium intake. In a study of calcium intake in individuals (56,58), no evidence of a relationship between cortical thickness and calcium intake was observed. In addition, results of clinical trials testing the efficacy of calcium supplementation in protecting against further bone loss in postmenopausal women have been contradictory (7,8,72,130,146), and at most suggest that if there is a beneficial effect from calcium, it is likely to be considerably less than that of estrogens.

A protective effect of fluoride has also been postulated. When fluoride is deposited in bone, the fluoride ion replaces the hydroxyl radical in hydroxyapatite to form fluorapatite at the surface of the crystals of bone salt. This substitution decreases the surface area, solubility, and chemical activity of the bone mineral, thus making it more stable (121,169). If administered for sufficiently long periods, fluoride has been reported to result in positive calcium balance in patients with osteoporosis, producing increases in bone mineralization and accretion rates (23,33,64,81, 91,124,132,133). It is therefore felt that perhaps fluoride could also protect against bone loss in healthy people. Epidemiologic studies to determine whether fluoride in drinking water does protect against osteoporosis have yielded conflicting results. The prevalence of osteoporosis based on radiographic findings was found to be higher in low-fluoride than in high-fluoride areas of North Dakota (24), and lower in a town in England where 1 ppm fluoride had been added to the water supply than in a comparison community with negligible amounts of fluoride in the water (15). However, no change was seen in the incidence of femoral fracture in women 60 years of age and older in a New York county before and after fluoridation of the water supply (61). In another study, lower death rates from falls were not found in localities with added fluorides compared to those with minimal fluoride, but rates were low in naturally fluoridated areas (76). It is thus possible that relatively high levels of fluorides over relatively long periods of time may be needed for a protective effect to be detectable. Animal experiments provide confirmatory evidence for this possibility, since they indicate that a certain dosage of fluoride must be reached before fluoride is protective (91,142,157).

Adequate amounts of vitamin D either from diet or from exposure to sunlight have been considered to have a protective effect, but definitive evidence is lacking (1,29,45,46,161). One investigator (112) reported that calcium absorption, which is diminished in older people (28), increases if vitamin D is administered in small doses, but it is far from established that diminished calcium absorption is a cause of osteoporosis.

Finally, a possible protective effect of physical activity against osteoporosis has been hypothesized. Severe or prolonged immobilization does result in disruption of bone formation (8,59,70,82), but the effect of mild or moderate immobilization is not known. Also, the possibility of a reduced risk among physically active healthy individuals has not been adequately studied. Differences in degree of physical activity among individuals in different countries have been postulated to be responsible for the varying incidence rates for fractures (31,119), but of course many other reasons could explain these international variations. One small prospective study (13) among postmenopausal women reported increases in total body calcium in an exercising group compared to a nonexercising group, but bone mineral content and total body potassium did not differ in the two groups. Thus, the role of physical exercise in the etiology of osteoporosis remains uncertain. However, further study is warranted since there are various mechanisms whereby physical activity could exert a protective effect, including a direct neural influence on bone, vascular and blood flow changes, and mechanical stress and strain resulting from the exercise (13).

Summary

Some risk factors for osteoporosis have been established, including sex, age, and race. Estrogen replacement therapy is undoubtedly protective, but many details remain to be learned about this relationship, including the importance of how close to menopause estrogen administration is started, the effect of the dose and duration of use, and the issue of how rapidly and to what extent bone loss continues after cessation of use. Obesity may also be protective, but more needs to be learned about the mechanism. Finally, more epidemiologic studies of the role of diet and physical activity are needed. Difficult though such studies may be, at least large associations between these factors and osteoporosis should be detectable.

OSTEOMALACIA AND RICKETS

In osteomalacia, normal bone is replaced through the usual mechanism of resorption and formation by nonmineralized osteoid. The total volume of bone is unchanged, but the mineral content is depleted because of lowered concentration of calcium or phosphorus in the body fluids as a result of impaired absorption from the gastrointestinal tract. Unlike osteoporosis, there is no interference with organic matrix formation. The pathogenesis and course of rickets is similar to that of osteomalacia, except that the former occurs only in growing bone and the latter in adult bone.

Absorption of calcium into the body requires vitamin D, which may be obtained from the diet or synthesized in the body by the action of sunlight on the skin. Deficiency of vitamin D leads to osteomalacia or rickets, depending on the age group. Signs and symptoms of osteomalacia and rickets include generalized pain or achiness, muscular weakness, tenderness over the long bones, skeletal deformity, a waddling gait, and bands of decalcification on the surface of the bone. The process may be reversed by vitamin D supplementation in the diet.

Diagnosis of osteomalacia and rickets may be made on the basis of clinical signs and symptoms, biochemical measures of serum calcium, serum phosphorous, and serum alkaline phosphatase, and radiographic findings. However, these methods do not have a high degree of accuracy (14,36,48,49,60) and it is often difficult to differentiate between osteomalacia and osteoporosis. Bone biopsy, which is necessary for accurate diagnosis (14,19,107), is obviously not a practical diagnostic tool in epidemiologic studies, so that most epidemiologic surveys necessarily rely on one or more of the less accurate methods. Consequently, most prevalence estimates are of limited value. The only report on the occurrence of osteomalacia that employed histologic diagnosis stated that 4 percent of 100 consecutive admissions to a geriatric unit in Scotland had the disease (14).

Despite these diagnostic problems, the major risk factors for osteomalacia and rickets are so obvious that they have been known for some time. Vitamin D deficiency in the diet has been identified as one of the basic causes of osteomalacia and rickets (16,20,40,43,102,139,156, 160,162,167) and lack of exposure to sunlight as the other (2,26,71,118,137,140). The ultraviolet radiation in sunlight brings about the synthesis of vitamin D in the skin, thereby protecting against osteomalacia and rickets. Vitamin D deficiency in the diet and lack of exposure to sunlight explain most of the other characteristics of the epidemiology of rickets and osteomalacia.

Osteomalacia and rickets are uncommon in continental Western Europe, where diet and exposure to sunlight are generally adequate, but these diseases are sometimes seen in the British Isles, probably because in Britain there is less exposure to sunlight than elsewhere in Europe (68,102,114,167). In the United States, where milk is routinely fortified with vitamin D, the disease is very rare, except perhaps among the elderly.

In other parts of the world such as Ethiopia (106), Pakistan (126), Iran (141), and India (4,32,95), osteomalacia and rickets are important problems. Estimates of prevalence in these areas range from 1 to 60 percent, but because different diagnostic procedures are used, exact prevalence figures are not meaningful. Inadequate diet obviously occurs among some segments of the population in these areas. In addition, even though there is an abundance of sunshine in a country such as India, the amount to which children and women are exposed may be reduced by the covering of the body with clothes while outdoors, the tendency to spend most time indoors, and the dirt and smoke in the atmosphere of the large cities. The extra pigment in the skin of most of the population of the area also reduces the extent of formation of vitamin D in the skin (4).

Prevalence rates are high among Asian immigrants in England, where it has been found that 10 to 24 percent of recent immigrants are affected (52,122). In all likelihood these high rates are attributable to the tendency of the migrants to continue to have diets low in vitamin D, and to have diminished formation of vitamin D in the skin because of the reduced amount of sunlight in the British Isles (122). In Scotland both clinical and subclinical rickets are more common among immigrant Asian children than among immigrant African, immigrant Chinese, or native Scottish children (60). However, rickets is still seen even among some of the native white children because of inadequate dietary vitamin D (37,134).

The age groups most frequently reported to have rickets or osteomalacia are children, women of childbearing years, and the elderly. Newborn infants born to healthy mothers have enough vitamin D for the first few months of life, but if sufficient vitamin D is not available after this time, calcium and phosphorus absorption from the intestinal tract is reduced; this affects the amount of calcium deposited in the growing bone, and rickets results. Women of childbearing age are thought to be at high risk because of pregnancy and lactation (50), although osteomalacia is also seen in nulliparous women of childbearing age (160). Women who bear several children at frequent intervals and who nurse them in between may lose considerable calcium and phosphorus while nursing; it is in this situation that osteomalacia may occur (3).

It is believed that geriatric populations are highly susceptible to the disease because of poor diets, lack of sunlight, and difficulty in absorbing fat-soluble vitamin D (30), and that much osteomalacia in the elderly passes unnoticed or misdiagnosed (1,122). Some investigators feel that the high prevalence of fractures following minimal trauma in the elderly is due to osteomalacia as well as to osteoporosis. Using iliac crest biopsies, two studies have found that the percentage of osteoid is greater in patients with proximal femoral fractures than in fracture-free patients (1,49). However, others have reported only small differences between fracture patients and others in osteoid content, unless there has been gastrectomy or a malabsorption syndrome (69,74,78,140).

Other aspects of dietary practices that have received some attention are phytate and fiber intake. Phytate, which occurs in high concentration in wholemeal wheat flour, impairs calcium absorption from the intestine by precipitating an insoluble calcium salt and binding it into a calcium-phytic acid complex (166). The leavening process reduces the phytate in bread, but many Indians use unleavened chupatty as a dietary mainstay. A few investigators have found that persons with osteomalacia eat more chupatty flour than people without osteomalacia, and that a chupatty-free diet reverses the biochemical abnormalities seen (42,51). However, others have observed no differences in phytate intake between cases with osteomalacia and controls (160,162). Reinhold (131) postulated that it is the high fiber in chupatties, not the phytate, which is detrimental to calcium absorption; the suggested mechanism is the metal-binding action of the fiber, which increases fecal losses of calcium, magnesium, and zinc. These relationships require further study.

Surgery of the digestive tract, particularly gastrectomy, can cause osteomalacia because of the resulting impaired absorption. For instance, gastrectomy patients in a twenty-year follow-up study had four times as many fractures associated with minimal or moderate trauma as did persons from the general population of their age, sex, and area of residence, thus supporting the hypothesis that gastrectomy increases the risk for osteomalacia, which in turn increases the risk for fractures (110). Osteomalacia has been found in 5 to 35 percent of postsurgical patients (36,44,66,116), although it is easily treated with vitamin D supplementation (105).

A genetic predisposition to osteomalacia has also been postulated (41,54), but the evidence for this is not strong. Heredity is not likely to be as important an etiologic agent as diet, sunlight, and, less frequently, surgery.

In summary, osteomalacia is rare in countries where people have access to adequate supplies of vitamin D, either from exposure to sunlight or in their diets. The relative importance of diet and sunlight in preventing osteomalacia has not been well studied, but it is likely that either of them in sufficient amounts may provide enough vitamin D to protect against the disease. The more minor reported associations of chupatty and fiber with osteomalacia are at present primarily speculative.

PAGET'S DISEASE OF BONE

Paget's disease of bone (also called osteitis deformans) is characterized by excessive resorption and subsequent excessive formation of bone, culminating in a "mosaic" pattern of normally parallel bone fibers associated with extensive local vascularity and increased fibrous tissue in adjacent marrow (84). This increased metabolic activity enlarges and softens the bone. The disease may occur in any bone, but most often affects the axial skeleton, especially the spine, femur, skull, sacrum, sternum, and pelvis (144). Paget's disease can be monostotic (occurring in only one bone) or polyostotic (occurring in several bones). It is often symptomless, but may produce bone pain and, in advanced or extensive cases, causes skeletal deformities in which the long bones become bowed, the skull enlarged, and vertebrae compressed. Pathologic fractures of affected bones are common, especially in the femur and tibia, and hearing loss frequently occurs when the skull is involved. Paget's disease is associated with an increased risk of primary bone tumors, including osteosarcomas, fibrosarcomas, chondrosarcomas, and benign and malignant giant cell tumors. From 7 to 22 percent of patients with polyostotic Paget's disease develop sarcomas, although the percentage is much lower among those with monostotic disease (65,147). Of bone tumors developing in persons over 40 years of age, up to 30 percent are in bones affected by Paget's disease (123). In the elderly the percentage is even higher. Other systemic complications may also occur that involve the musculoskeletal, nervous, cardiovascular, and endocrine systems.

Various drugs that suppress bone resorption are used to treat symptomatic cases. Prognosis is variable, depending on the number and location of affected bones. Many people live out their lives without knowing they have the disease; others have considerable pain and become deformed, and some die from the complications.

Paget's disease may be diagnosed after a person complains of pain or deformity, but it is often an incidental finding on X-rays taken for other purposes. Serum alkaline phosphatase concentrations are commonly used to confirm X-ray findings, but with disease of limited extent, these concentrations may be normal. Then, bone biopsies or scans may be used.

Paget's disease has been found in some studies to occur with about equal frequency in men and women and in others to be slightly more common in males; it is seldom found in people under 40 years of age (3,35,120,144). Because of the frequent lack of symptoms and the need for invasive procedures for accurate diagnosis, epidemiologic studies of Paget's disease are difficult to conduct, and only a few have been done. Consequently, most knowledge of the population distribution of Paget's disease comes from postmortem investigations and from studies based on X-rays taken for other reasons.

Surveys in England and Germany have estimated the prevalence rate of Paget's disease to be 3 to 4 percent in autopsied individuals over 40 years of age and about 9 to 10 percent in those who died at age 85 years and over (35,144). Pygott (125) found evidence of Paget's disease in 3.5 percent of X-rays which included the lumbar spine and pelvis in 9775 patients over 45 years of age in London. Comparison of blacks and whites suggest no significant differences in prevalence rates (86,138).

Clinical impressions suggest that the prevalence of Paget's disease varies greatly from one geographic location to another. It is considered relatively common in Britain, most of continental Europe, and the United States, but appears to occur less frequently in Scandinavia (149). Cases have rarely been reported in Africa and Asia, but this may be because many asymptomatic cases remain undiagnosed and because the populations in these areas are relatively young. That caution must be used in making geographic and temporal comparisons is emphasized by Porretta et al. (120), who believed that an increase in the proportion of cases of Paget's disease among admissions to the Mayo Clinic from 1 per 16,000 admissions in 1921 to 1 per 900 admissions in the 1950s was attributable to cases missed in the earlier period. Improved diagnostic methods and greater awareness by physicians have undoubtedly increased the frequency with which Paget's disease is diagnosed.

The etiology of Paget's disease is essentially unknown, but research into a recently developed theory that a virus with a long incubation period is involved shows some promising results. Intranuclear inclusions similar to those found in cells affected by subacute sclerosing panencephalitis (SSPE), which is believed to be caused by a virus with a long incubation period, were found by investigators in both France and Los Angeles to be present in osteoclasts from bone samples taken from patients with Paget's disease, but not in samples from patients with other metabolic bone diseases (103,127–129,148). Also, the investigators from France (127,128) have subsequently suggested on the basis of immunofluorescent techniques that the measles virus or a measles-related virus is the responsible agent, but this was not found by the Los Angeles group (104), who did, however, note that the immunofluorescent techniques were positive for the respiratory syncytial virus. Singer and Mills (148) have suggested that the disease may be a form of a benign tumor that becomes malignant in some cases, possibly through a slow-virus infection.

Observations of diets of horses developing "big head" disease, of the apparent international geographic variation in prevalence rates of Paget's disease in humans, and of the improvement of symptoms in affected patients after phosphorus levels are reduced, have led to the hypothesis that high levels of dietrary phosphorus may be involved in the etiology (3). However, to date this hypothesis has apparently not been tested. Also, it has been noted in Britain that the geographic distributions of Paget's disease and rickets are similar, suggesting a possible relationship between Vitamin D deficiency and subsequent development of Paget's disease (21).

Paget's disease can occur in several members of a family, leading to the speculation that it is genetic in origin (47,55). This is of course only one possible explanation of the familial aggregation, if the occurrence of multiple cases within families is indeed greater than would be expected by chance. It has been suggested that in some families Paget's disease may be inherited as an autosomal dominant trait linked to the HLA histocompatibility antigen without maintaining significant linkage disequilibrium (53), but since this observation was based on three generations of only three families, further evaluation is needed. McKusick (97) has argued that the disease results from an inborn error of connective-tissue synthesis. However, Singer and Mills (148) point out the Paget's disease is probably not an heritable generalized disorder of connective tissue because it is most often localized in the skeleton. Furthermore, Melick and Martin (101) note that if the disease is genetically caused, there should be concordance in identical twins, and that only five identical twin pairs with both members affected have been reported.

Other suggested etiologic factors are mechanical stress to bone, autoimmune dysfunctions, vascular disorders, and hormonal deficiencies, but there is little support for these theories (148). The most promising area for both epidemiologic and laboratory research appears to be further exploration of the possibility of a slow-virus etiology.

REFERENCES

1. Aaron, J. E., Gallagher, J. C., Anderson, J., Stasiak, L., Longton, E. B., Nordin, B. E. C., and Nicholson, M. 1974. "Frequency of osteomalacia and osteoporosis in fractures of the proximal femur." *Lancet* 1:229–233.
2. ———, Gallagher, J. C., and Nordin, B. E. C. 1974. "Seasonal variation of histological osteomalacia in femoral-neck fractures." *Lancet* 2:84–85.
3. Aegerter, E., and Kirkpatrick, J. A., Jr. 1964. *Orthopaedic Diseases.* Philadelphia: Saunders.
4. Agrawal, J. R., Sheth, S. C., and Tibrewala, N. S. 1969. "Rickets—A study of 300 cases." *Indian Pediat.* 6:792–798.
5. Aitken, J. M., Hart, D. M., and Lindsay, R. 1973. "Oestrogen replacement therapy for prevention of osteoporosis after oophorectomy." *Brit. Med. J.* 3:515–518.
6. ———, Hart, D. M., Lindsay, R., Anderson, J. B., Smith, D. A., and Wilson, G. M. 1976. "Prevention of bone loss following oophorectomy in premenopausal women." *Israel J. Med. Sci.* 12:607–614.
7. Albanese, A. A. 1978. "Calcium nutrition in the elderly." *Postgrad. Med.* 63:167–172.
8. ———, Edelson, A. H., Lorenze, E. J., Woodhull, M. L., and Wein, E. H. 1975. "Problems of bone health in the elderly." *N.Y. State J. Med.* 75:326–336.
9. Albright, F., Bloomberg, E., and Smith, P. H. 1940. "Post-menopausal osteoporosis." *Trans. Ass. Am. Phys.* 55:298–305.

10. Albright, J. A., and Skinner, H. C. W. 1979. "Bone: Remodeling dynamics." In *The Scientific Basis of Orthopaedics.* J. A. Albright and R. A. Brand, eds. New York: Appleton, pp. 185–229.

11. Alffram, P-A. 1964. "An epidemiological study of cervical and trochanteric fractures of the femur in an urban population." *Acta Orthop. Scand. Suppl.* 65:1–109.

12. Alhava, E. M., and Puittinen, J. 1973. "Fractures of the upper end of the femur as an index of senile osteoporosis in Finland." *Ann. Clin. Res.* 5:398–403.

13. Aloia, J. F., Cohn, S. H., Ostuni, J. A., Cane, R., and Ellis, K. 1978. "Prevention of involutional bone loss by exercise." *Ann. Int. Med.* 89:356–358.

14. Anderson, I., Campbell, A. E. R., Dunn, A., and Runciman, J. B. M. 1966. "Osteomalacia in elderly women." *Scott. Med. J.* 11:429–435.

15. Ansell, B. M., and Lawrence, J. S. 1965. "Fluoridation and the rheumatic diseases. A comparison of rheumatism in Watford and Leigh." *Ann. Rheum. Dis.* 25:67–75.

16. Arneil, G. G. 1975. "Nutritional rickets in children in Glasgow." *Proc. Nutr. Soc.* 34:101–109.

17. ———, and Crosbie, J. C. 1963. "Infantile rickets returns to Glasgow." *Lancet* 2:423–425.

18. Atkinson, P. J. 1965. "Changes in resorption spaces in femoral cortical bone with age." *J. Path. Bact.* 89:173–178.

19. Avioli, L. V. 1979. "Management of osteomalacia." *Hosp. Prac.* 14:109–114.

20. Awwar, M. 1978. "Nutritional hypovitaminosis-D and the genesis of osteomalacia in the elderly." *J. Amer. Geriat. Soc.* 26:309–317.

21. Barker, D. J. P., and Gardner, M. J. 1974. "Distribution of Paget's disease in England, Wales, and Scotland and a possible relationship with Vitamin D deficiency in childhood." *Brit. J. Prev. Soc. Med.* 28:226–232.

22. Bauer, G. C. H. 1960. "Epidemiology of fractures in aged persons." *Clin. Orthop.* 17:219–225.

23. Bernstein, D. S., and Cohen, P. 1967. "Use of sodium fluoride in the treatment of osteoporosis." *J. Clin. End.* 27:197–210.

24. ———, Sadowsky, N., Hegsted, D. M., Guri, C. D., and Stare, F. J. 1966. "Prevalence of osteoporosis in high- and low-fluoride areas in North Dakota." *J. Amer. Med. Ass.* 198:499–504.

25. Bollet, A. J., Engh, G., and Parson, W. 1965. "Epidemiology of osteoporosis." *Arch. Int. Med.* 116:191–194.

26. Boyle, I. T. 1974. "Vitamin D—An old hormone rediscovered." *Scott. Med. J.* 19:247–249.

27. Buhr, A. J., and Cooke, A. M. 1959. "Fracture patterns." *Lancet* 1:531–536.

28. Bullamore, J. R., Gallagher, J. C., Wilkinson, R., and Nordin, B. E. C. 1970. "Effect of age on calcium absorption." *Lancet* 2:535–537.

29. Burton, J. L., Ensell, F. J., Leach, J. F., and Hali, K. A. 1975. "Atmospheric ozone and femoral fractures." *Lancet* 1:795–796.

30. Chalmers, G. L. 1978. "Disorders of bone." *Practitioner* 220:711–721.

31. Chalmers, J., and Ho, K. C. 1970. "Geographic variation in senile osteoporosis." *J. Bone Jt. Surg. (Brit.)* 52:667–675.

32. Chaudhuri, M. K. 1975. "Nutritional profile of Calcutta pre-school children II. Clinical observations." *Indian J. Med. Res.* 63:189–195.

33. Cohen, P., and Gardner, F. H. 1966. "Induction of skeletal fluorosis in two common demineralizing disorders." *J. Amer. Med. Ass.* 195:962–963.

34. Cohn, S. H., Abesamis, C., Yasumura, S., Aloia, J. F., Zanzi, I., and Ellis, K. J. 1977. "Comparative skeletal mass and radial bone mineral content in Black and White women." *Metabolism* 26:171–178.

35. Collins, D. H. 1956. "Paget's disease of bone. Incidence of subclinical forms." *Lancet* 2:51–57.
36. Compston, J. E., Ayers, A. B., Horton, L. W. L., Tighe, J. R., and Creamer, B. 1978. "Osteomalacia after small-intestinal resection." *Lancet* 1:9–12.
37. Cooke, W. T., Swan, C. H. J., Asquith, P., Melikian, V., and McFeely, W. E. 1973. "Serum alkaline phosphatase and rickets in urban schoolchildren." *Brit. Med. J.* 1:324–327.
38. Davis, M. E., Lanzl, L. H., and Cox, A. B. 1970. "Detection, prevention, and retardation of menopausal osteoporosis." *Obstet. Gyn.* 36:187–198.
39. ———, Strandjord, N. M., and Lanzl, L. H. 1966. "Estrogens and the aging process." *J. Amer. Med. Ass.* 196:219–224.
40. Dent, C. E., and Smith, R. 1969. "Nutritional osteomalacia." *Quart. J. Med.* 38:195–209.
41. Doxiadis, S., Angelis, C., Karatzas, P., Vrettos, C., and Lapatsanis, P. 1976. "Genetic aspects of nutritional rickets." *Arch Dis. Child.* 51:83–90.
42. Dunnigan, M. G., McIntosh, W. B., and Ford, J. A. 1976. "Rickets in Asian immigrants." *Lancet* 1:1346.
43. Dwyer, J. T., Dietz, W. H., Hass, G., and Suskind, R. 1979. "Risk of nutritional rickets among vegetarian children." *Amer. J. Dis. Child* 133:134–140.
44. Eddy, R. L. 1971. "Metabolic bone disease after gastrectomy." *Amer. J. Med.* 50:442–447.
45. Eddy, T. P. 1973. "Deaths from domestic falls and fractures." *Brit. J. Prev. Soc. Med.* 26:173–179.
46. Engh, G., Bollet, A. J., Hardin, G., and Parson, W. 1968. "Epidemiology of osteoporosis: II Incidence of hip fractures in mental institutions." *J. Bone Jt. Surg. (Amer.)* 50:557–562.
47. Evens, R. G., and Bartter, F. C. 1968. "The hereditary aspects of Paget's disease (osteitis deformans)." *J. Amer. Med. Ass.* 205:900–902.
48. Exton-Smith, A. N., Hodkinson, H. M., and Stanton, B. R. 1966. "Nutrition and metabolic bone disease in old age." *Lancet* 2:999–1000.
49. Faccini, J. M., Exton-Smith, A. N., and Boyde, A. 1976. "Disorders of bone and fracture of the femoral neck." *Lancet* 1:1089–1095.
50. Felton, D. J. C., and Stone, W. D. 1966, "Osteomalacia in Asian immigrants during pregnancy." *Brit. Med. J.* 1:1521–1522.
51. Ford, J. A., Colhoun, E. M., McIntosh, W. B., and Dunnigan, M. G. 1972. "Biochemical response of late rickets and osteomalacia to a chupatty-free diet."
52. ——— et al. 1972. "Rickets and osteomalacia in the Glasgow Pakistani community, 1961–71." *Brit. Med. J.* 2:677–680.
53. Fotino, M., Haymovits, A., and Falk, C. T. 1977. "Evidence for linkage between HLA and Paget's disease." *Transplant. Proc.* 11:1867–1868.
54. Frymoyer, J. W., and Hodgkin, W. 1977. "Adult-onset vitamin D-resistant hypophosphatemic osteomalacia." *J. Bone Jt. Surg. (Amer.)* 59:101–106.
55. Galbraith, H. J-B., Evans, E. C., and Lacey, J. 1977. "Paget's disease of bone: A clinical and genetic study." *Postgrad. Med. J.* 53:35–39.
56. Garn, S. M. 1970. *The Earlier Gain and Later Loss of Cortical Bone in Nutritional Perspective.* Springfield: Ill.: Charles C. Thomas.
57. ———. 1975. "Bone loss and aging." In *Physiology and Pathology of Human Aging.* R. Goldman, ed. New York: Academic Press. pp. 39–57.
58. ———, Rohmann, C. G., and Wagner, B. 1967. "Bone loss as a general phenomenon in man." *Fed. Proc.* 26:1729–1736.
59. Geiser, M., and Trueta, J. 1958. "Muscle action, bone rarefaction, and bone formation." *J. Bone Jt. Surg. (Brit.)* 40:282–310.

60. Goel, K. M., Logan, R. W., Arneil, G. C., Sweet, E. M., Warren, J. M., and Shanks, R. A. 1976. "Fluoride and subclinical rickets among immigrant children in Glasgow." *Lancet* 1:1141–1145.
61. Goggin, J. E., Hacklon, W., Hambly, G. S., and Hoveland, J. R. 1965. "Incidence of femoral fractures in post-menopausal women." *Pub. Hlth. Rep.* 80:1005–1010.
62. Goldsmith, W. F., and Johnston, J. O. 1975. "Bone mineral effects of oral contraceptives, pregnancy, and lactation." *J. Bone Jt. Surg. (Amer.)* 57:657–668.
63. Grodin, J. M., Siiteri, P. K., and MacDonald, P. C. 1973. "Source of estrogen production in post-menopausal women." *J. Clin. Endocr. Metab.* 36:207–214.
64. Gron, P., McCann, H. G., and Bernstein, D. 1966. "Effect of fluoride on human osteoporotic bone mineral." *J. Bone Jt. Surg. (Amer.)* 48:892–898.
65. Harris, S. 1978, "Paget disease of bone." *Western J. Med.* 129:210–224.
66. Harvald, B., Krogsgaard, A. R., and Lous, P. 1962. "Calcium deficiency following partial gastrectomy." *Acta Med. Scand.* 172:497–503.
67. Hernberg, C. A. 1960. "Treatment of postmenopausal osteoporosis with oestrogens and androgens." *Acta Endocr.* 34:51–59.
68. Hodgkin, P., Hine, P. M., Kay, G. H., and Lumb, G. A. 1973. "Vitamin-D deficiency in Asians at home and in Britain." *Lancet* 2:167–172.
69. Hodkinson, H. M. 1971. "Fracture of the femoral neck in the elderly, assessment of the role of osteomalacia." *Geront. Clin.* 13:153–158.
70. Hodkinson, H. M., and Brain, A. T. 1967. "Unilateral osteoporosis in longstanding hemiplegia in the elderly." *J. Amer. Geriat. Soc.* 15:59–64.
71. ———, Round, P., Stanton, B. R., and Morgan, C. 1973. "Sunlight, vitamin D, and osteomalacia in the elderly." *Lancet* 1:910–912.
72. Horsman, A., Nordin, B. E. C., Gallagher, J. C., Kirby, P. A., Milner, R. H., and Simpson, M. 1976. "Observations on sequential changes in bone mass in postmenopausal women: A controlled trial of oestrogen and calcium therapy." *Calc. Tissue Res.* 22:217–224.
73. Hui, S. L. 1979. "Statistical modeling of longitudinal data applied to the change of bone mass in postmenopausal women." Thesis, Ph.D., Epidemiology and Public Health, Yale University.
74. Hulth, A. G., Nilsson, B. E., Westlin, N. E., Wiklund, P. E. 1979. "Bone biopsy in women with spinal osteoporosis." *Acta Med. Scand.* 206:205–206.
75. Hutchinson, T. A., Polansky, S. M., and Feinstein, A. R. 1979. "Postmenopausal oestrogens protect against fractures of hip and distal radius: a case-control study." *Lancet* 2:705–709.
76. Iskrant, A. P. 1968. "The etiology of fractured hips in females." *Amer. J. Publ. Hlth.* 58:485–490.
77. ———, and Smith, R. W. 1969. "Osteoporosis in women 45 years and over related to subsequent fracture." *Publ Hlth. Rep.* 84:33–38.
78. Jenkins, D. H. R., Roberts, J. G., Webster, D., and Williams, E. O. 1973. "Osteomalacia in elderly patients with fracture of the femoral neck." *J. Bone Jt. Surg. (Brit.)* 55:575–580.
79. Johnson, R. E., and Specht, E. E. 1979. "The risk of hip fracture in postmenopausal females with and without estrogen drug exposure." American Public Health Association, New York. Paper presented to Epidemiology Section.
80. Jowsey, J., and Raisz, L. G. 1968. "Experimental osteoporosis and parathyroid activity." *Endocrinology* 82:384–396.
81. ———, Schenk, R. K., and Reutter, F. W. 1968. "Some results of the effect of fluoride on bone tissue in osteoporosis." *J. Clin. End.* 28:869–874.
82. Kesson, C. M., Morris, N., and McCutcheon, A. 1947. "Generalized osteoporosis in old age." *Ann. Rheum. Dis.* 6:146–161.

83. Knowelden, J., Buhr, A. J., and Dunbar, O. 1964. "Incidence of fractures in persons over 35 years of age." *Brit. J. Prev. Soc. Med.* 18:130–141.
84. Krane, S. M. 1977. "Paget's disease of bone." *Clin. Orthop.* 127:24–36
85. Kreiger, N. 1980. "An epidemiologic study of hip fracture in postmenopausal women." Thesis, Ph.D., Epidemiology and Public Health, Yale University.
86. Lawrence, J. S. 1970. "Paget's disease in population samples." (Abstract) *Ann. Rheum. Dis.* 29:562.
87. Leitch, I. H., Knowelden, J., and Seddon, H. J. 1964. "Incidence of fractures, particularly of the neck of the femur, in patients in mental hospitals." *Brit. J. Prev. Soc. Med.* 18:142–145.
88. Levine, S., Makin, M., Menczel, J., Robin, G., Naor, E., and Steinberg, R. 1970. "Incidence of fractures of the proximal end of the femur in Jerusalem." *J. Bone Jt. Surg. (Amer.)* 52:1193–1202.
89. Lindsay, R. Hart, D. M., MacLean, A., Clark, A. C., Kraszewski, A., and Garwood, J. 1978. "Bone response to termination of oestrogen treatment." *Lancet* 1:1325–1327.
90. ———, Hart, D. M., Purdie, D., Ferguson, M. M., Clark, A. C., and Kraszewski, A. 1978. "Comparative effects of oestrogen and a progestogen on bone loss in post-menopausal women." *Clin. Sci. Molec. Med.* 54:193–195.
91. Lukert, B. P., Bolinger, R. E., and Meek, J. C. 1967. "Acute effect of fluoride on calcium dynamics in osteoporosis." *J. Clin. End.* 27:828–835.
92. MacDonald, P. C., and Siiteri, P. K. 1974. "The relationship between the extra-glandular production of estrone and the occurrence of endometrial neoplasia." *Gynec. Oncol.* 2:259–263.
93. Macuch, P., Kortus, J., Balazova, G., and Mayer, G. 1968. "Effects of sodium and hydrogen fluorides on the metabolism of fluorine, calcium, and phosphorus in rats." *Brit. J. Industr. Med.* 25:131–135.
94. Makin, M., Menczel, J., and Robin, G. 1970. "The incidence of fractures of the hip in Jerusalem (1957–1966) as an index of osteoporosis." In *Osteoporosis.* U.S. Barzel, ed. New York: Grune and Stratton. pp. 164–173.
95. Mankodi, N. A., Mankikar, A., Shiddhye, S., and Shah, P. M. 1974. "Rickets in pre-school age children in and around Bombay." *Trop. Geograph. Med.* 26:375–378.
96. Marshall, D. H., Horsman, A., and Nordin, B. E. C. 1977. "The prevention and management of postmenopausal osteoporosis." *Acta. Obstet. Gynec. Scand. Suppl.* 65:49–56.
97. McKusick, V. A. 1972. *Heritable Disorders of Connective Tissue.* St. Louis: The C. V. Mosby Co.
98. Meema, H. E., and Meema, S. 1968. "Prevention of postmenopausal osteoporosis by hormone treatment of the menopause." *Canad. Med. Ass. J.* 99:248–251.
99. ———, and Meema, S. 1974. "Involutional (physiologic) bone loss in women and the feasibility of preventing structural failure." *J. Am. Geriat. Soc.* 22:443–452.
100. ———, and Meema, S. 1976. "Menopausal bone loss and estrogen replacement." *Israeli J. Med. Sci.* 12:601–606.
101. Melick, R. A., and Martin, T. J. 1975. "Paget's disease in identical twins." *Aust. N. Z. J. Med.* 5:564–565.
102. Miller, C. G., and Chutkan, W. 1976. "Vitamin-D deficiency rickets in Jamaican children." *Arch. Dis. Child.* 51:214–218.
103. Mills, B. G., and Singer, F. R. 1976. "Nuclear inclusions in Paget's disease of bone." *Science* 199:201–202.
104. ———, Singer, F. R., Weiner, L. P., and Holst, P. A. 1980. "Immunohistological evidence of respiratory syncytial virus in Paget's disease of bone." (Abstract) *Calc. Tissue Res.* 31:64.

105. Morgan, D. B., Paterson, C. R., Pulvertabt, C. N., Woods, C. G., and Fourman, P. 1965. "Osteomalacia after gastrectomy. A response to very small doses of vitamin D." *Lancet* 2:1089–1091.
106. Mumdziev, N., 1968. "Rachitis in children up to 2 years of age in Addis Abeba (Ethiopia) and some peculiarities in its clinical picture." *Folia Medica (Plovdiv)* 10:198–201.
107. Mundy, G. R. 1978. "Differential diagnosis of osteopenia." *Hosp. Pract.* 13:65–72.
108. Nachtigall, L. E., Nachtigall, R. H., Nachtigall, R. D., and Beckman, E. M. 1979. "Estrogen replacement therapy I: A 10-year prospective study on the relationship to osteoporosis." *Obstet. Gynec.* 53:277–281.
109. Newton-John, H. F., and Morgan, D. B. 1970. "The loss of bone with age, osteoporosis and fractures." *Clin. Orthop.* 71:229–252.
110. Nilsson, B. E., and Westlin, N. E. 1971. "The fracture incidence after gastrectomy." *Acta. Chir. Scand.* 137:533–534.
111. Nordin. B. E. C. 1966. "International patterns of osteoporosis." *Clin. Orthop.* 45:17–20.
112. ———. 1971. "Clinical significance and pathogenesis of osteoporosis." *Brit. Med. J.* 1:571–576.
113. ———, MacGregor, J., and Smith, D. A. 1966. "The incidence of osteoporosis in normal women: Its relationship to age and the menopause." *Quart. J. Med.* 35:25–38.
114. O'Hara-May, J., and Widdowson, E. M. 1976. "Diets and living conditions of Asian boys in Coventry with and without signs of rickets." *Brit. J. Nutrit.* 36:23–36.
115. Paganini-Hill, A., Ross, R. K., Gerkins, V. R., and Mack, T. M. 1979. "Menopausal estrogen use and hip fractures." (Abstract) *Cancer Treatment Rep.* 63:1210.
116. Parfitt, A. M., Miller, M. J., Frame, B., Villanueva, A. R., Rao, D. S., Oliver, I., and Thomson, D. L. 1978. "Metabolic bone disease after intestinal bypass for treatment of obesity." *Ann. Int. Med.* 89:193–199.
117. Paterson, C. R. 1978. "Calcium requirements in man: a critical review." *Postgrad. Med. J.* 54:244–248.
118. Pittet, P. G., Davie, M., and Lawson, D. E. M. 1979. "Role of nutrition in the development of osteomalacia in the elderly." *Nutr. Metab.* 23:109–116.
119. Pogrund, H., Makin, M., Robin, G., Menczel, J., and Steinberg, R. 1977. "The epidemiology of femoral neck fractures in Jerusalem." *Clin. Orthop.* 122:141–146.
120. Porretta, C. A., Dahlin, D. C., and James, J. H. 1957. "Sarcoma in Paget's disease of bone." *J. Bone Jt. Surg. (Amer.)* 39:1314–1329.
121. Posner, A. A., Eanes, E. D., Harper, R. A., and Zipkin, I. 1963. "X-ray diffraction analysis of the effect of fluoride on human bone apatite." *Arch. Oral Biol.* 8:549–570.
122. Preece, M. A., Tomlinson, S., Ribot, C. A., Pietrek, J., Korn, H. T., Davies, D. M., Ford, J. A., Dunnigan, M. G., and O'Riordan, J. L. H. 1975. "Studies of vitamin D deficiency in man." *Quart. J. Med.* 44:575–589.
123. Price, C. H. G. 1962. "Incidence of osteogenic sarcoma in southwest England and its relationship to Paget's disease of bone." *J. Bone Jt. Surg. (Brit.)* 44:366–376.
124. Purves, M. J. 1962. "Some effects of administering sodium fluoride to patients with Paget's disease." *Lancet* 2:1188–1189.
125. Pygott, F. 1957. "Paget's disease of bone. The radiological incidence." *Lancet* 1:1170–1171.

126. Rab, S. M., and Baseer, A. 1976. "Occult osteomalacia amongst healthy and pregnant women in Pakistan." *Lancet* 2:1211–1213.

127. Rebel, A., Baslé, M., Puupland, A., Kouyoumdjian, S., Filmon, R., and Leputezour, A. 1980. "Viral antigens in osteoclasts from Paget's disease of bone." *Lancet* 2:344–346.

128. ———, Baslé M., Puupland A., Malkani, K., Filmon, R., and Lepatezour, A. 1980. "Bone tissue in Paget's disease of bone." *Arth. Rheum.* 23:1104–1114.

129. ———, Malkani, K., Baslé, M., and Bregeon, C. 1976. "Osteoclast ultrastructure in Paget's disease." *Calcif. Tiss. Res.* 20:187–199.

130. Recker, R. R., Saville, P. D., and Heaney, R. P. 1977. "Effect of estrogens and calcium carbonate on bone loss in postmenopausal women." *Ann. Int. Med.* 87:649–655.

131. Reinhold, J. G. 1976. "Rickets in Asian immigrants." *Lancet* 2:1132–1133.

132. Rich, C., and Ensinck, J. 1961. "Effect of sodium fluoride on calcium metabolism in human beings." *Nature* 191:184–185.

133. ———, and Ivanovich, P. 1965. "Response to sodium fluoride in severe primary osteoporosis." *Ann. Intern. Med.* 63:1069–1074.

134. Richards, I. D. G., Sweet, E. M., and Arneil, G. C. 1968. "Infantile rickets persists in Glasgow." *Lancet* 1:803–805.

135. Riggs, B. L., Jowsey, J., Goldsmith, R. S., Kelly, P. J., Hoffman, D. L., and Arnaud, C. D. 1972. "Short-and long-term effects of estrogen and synthetic anabolic hormone in postmenopausal osteoporosis." *J. Clin. Invest.* 51:1659–1663.

136. ———, Jowsey, J., Kelly, P. J., and Arnaud, C. D. 1976. "Role of hormonal factors in the pathogenesis of postmenopausal osteoporosis." *Israeli J. Med. Sci.* 12:615–619.

137. Rizvi, S. N. A., Chawla, S. C., Sinha, S., Malhotra, P., Gulati, P. D., and Vaishnava, H. 1976. "Some observations on the prevalence of vitamin D deficiency rickets amongst families of osteomalacics." *J. Assoc. Physic. India* 24:833–838.

138. Rosenkrantz, J. A., Wolf, J., and Kaicher, J. J. 1952. "Paget's disease (osteitis deformans). Review of one hundred eleven cases." *A.M.A. Arch. Int. Med.* 90:610–633.

139. Ruck, N. 1974. "An individual dietary survey of schoolchildren in Birmingham." *Proc. Nutr. Soc.* 33:17A–18A.

140. Rush, J. H. 1977. "Osteomalacia in the elderly." *Aust. New Zeal. J. Surg.* 47:186–188.

141. Salimpour, R. 1975. "Rickets in Tehran. Study of 200 cases." *Arch. Dis. Child.* 50:63–66.

142. Saville, P. D. 1967. "Water fluoridation: Effect on bone fragility and skeletal calcium content in the rat." *J. Nutr.* 91:353–357.

143. ———, and Nilsson, B. E. R. 1966. "Height and weight in symptomatic postmenopausal osteoporosis." *Clin. Orthop.* 45:49–54.

144. Schmorl, G. 1932. "Uber Osteitis deformans Paget." *Arch. Path. Anat. Physiol.* 283:694–751.

145. Scott, S., Gray, D. H., and Stevenson, W. 1980. "The incidence of femoral neck fractures in New Zealand." *New Zeal. Med. J.* 91:6–9.

146. Shapiro, J., Moore, W. T., Jorgensen, H., Reid, J., Epps, C. H., and Whedon, D. 1975. "Osteoporosis." *Arch. Int. Med.* 135:563–567.

147. Singer, F. R. 1977. *Paget's Disease of Bone.* New York: Plenum.

148. ———, and Mills, B. G. 1977. "The etiology of Paget's disease of bone." *Clin. Orthop.* 127:37–42.

149. Sissons, H. A. 1966. "The epidemiology of Paget's disease." *Clin. Orthop.* 45:73–79.

150. Smith, R. W., and Rizek, J. 1966. "Epidemiological studies of osteoporosis in women of Puerto Rico and southeastern Michigan with special reference to age, race, national origin, and to other related or associated findings." *Clin. Orthop.* 45:31–48.

151. Solomon, G. F., Dickerson, W. J., and Eisenberg, E. 1960. "Psychologic and osteometabolic response to sex hormones in elderly osteoporotic women." *Geriatrics* 15:46–60.

152. Solomon, L. 1968. "Osteoporosis and fracture of the femoral neck in the South African Bantu." *J. Bone Jt. Surg. (Brit.)* 50:2–13.

153. Stevens, J., Freeman, P. A. Nordin, B. E.C., and Barnett, E. 1962. "The incidence of osteoporosis in patients with femoral neck fracture." *J. Bone Jt. Surg. (Brit.)* 44:520–527.

154. Stewart, I. M. 1955. "Fractures of the neck of the femur: Incidence and implications." *Brit. Med. J.* 1:698–701.

155. Strange, F. G. S. 1965. *The Hip.* London: Heinemann.

156. Swan, C. H. J., and Cooke, W. T. 1971. "Nutritional osteomalacia in immigrants in an urban community." *Lancet* 2:456–459.

157. Szob, Z., and Geisler, J. 1967. "Influence of fluoride ion on the calcification process in rat bone." *Acta Biochim. Polonica* 14:111–120.

158. Trotter, M., Broman, G. E, and Peterson, R. R. 1960. "Densities of bones of White and Negro skeletons." *J. Bone Jt. Surg. (Amer.)* 42:50–58.

159. Utian, W. H. 1971. "Oestrogens and osteoporosis." *S. Afr. Med.J.* 45:879–882.

160. Vaishnava, H., 1975. "Vitamin-D deficiency osteomalacia in northern India." *J. Assoc. Physicians India* 23:477–484.

161. Vaishnava, H., and Rizvi, S. N. A. 1974. "Frequency of osteomalacia and osteoporosis in fractures of proximal femur." *Lancet* 1:676–677.

162. ———, and Rizvi, S. N. A. 1967. "Osteomalacia in Northern India." *Brit. Med. J.* 1:112.

163. ———, and Rizvi, S. N. A. 1973. "Vitamin-D deficiency osteomalacia in Asians." *Lancet* 2:621–622.

164. Walker, A. R. P. 1972. "The human requirement of calcium: should low intakes be supplemented?" *Am. J. Clin. Nutr.* 25:518–530.

165. Weiss, N. S,. Ure, C. L., Ballard, J. H., Williams, A. R., and Daling, J. R. 1980. "Decreased risk of fractures of the hip and lower forearm with postmenopausal use of estrogen." *New Engl. J. Med.* 303:1195–1198.

166. Wills, M. R., Phillips, J. B., Day, R. C., and Bateman, E C. 1972. Phytic acid and nutritional rickets in immigrants," *Lancet* 1:771–773.

167. Wilson, D. C. 1931. "The incidence of osteomalacia and late rickets in Northern India." *Lancet* 2:10–12.

168. Wong, P. C. N. 1966. "Fracture epidemiology in a mixed southeast Asian community (Singapore)." *Clin. Orthop.* 45:55–61.

169. Young, R. A., Van Der Lugt, A., and Elliott, J. C. 1969. "Osteoporosis." *Nature* 223:729–730.

6 Conditions Affecting the Back and Neck

Pain in the back and in the neck are very common problems in Western countries, and are a major cause of morbidity, disability, limitation of activity, and economic loss. Nevertheless, relative to the magnitude of the problem, few epidemiologic studies have focused on back and neck problems. Another major difficulty in presenting material on these conditions is that most investigators have considered back or neck pain as a whole. Many different disease processes, each with specific etiologic characteristics, can result in low back or neck pain. In this chapter, therefore, studies will be emphasized that focus on specific conditions, such as prolapsed discs, degenerated discs, and spondylolisthesis. Other diseases that frequently affect the back, including osteoporosis, osteoarthrosis, ankylosing spondylitis, adolescent scoliosis and kyphosis, and spina bifida, are discussed elsewhere.

Before considering the individual diseases, however, some general aspects of low back pain, which is of major interest, and of neck pain, will be briefly reviewed, to the extent that available data permit. This is done because in a large proportion of cases of low back and neck pain, no definite diagnosis can be made, with the result that limiting the discussion to specific diseases would exclude the vast majority of people with low back and neck pain. This is illustrated in a study of acute low back pain seen by general practitioners in London, England (22), in which it was found that in 79 percent of first attacks of low back pain in men and in 89 percent in women, no specific reason for the pain could be identified (Table 6-1). Nevertheless, the symptom of low back pain is very frequent, and merits discussion, even though in the future it may become possible

Table 6-1 Percentage Distribution of Causes of First Episodes of Acute Low Back Pain Seen in General Practice, Southeast London, 1957–1960

Cause	Males	Females
Not known	79.3	88.8
Strain	10.9	4.3
Proved prolapsed disc	7.6	5.6
Other	2.1	1.2
Number of patients	184 ,	161

Source: Dillane et al. (22).

to subdivide the various types of low back pain to a greater extent than is currently possible.

BACK AND NECK PAIN: GENERAL ASPECTS

The importance of back and neck pain in both the general population and industrial populations has been well documented. Hult (43), for instance, found that 60 percent of Swedish males from the general population had at some time suffered from symptoms related to the low back, 16 percent had been incapacitated for periods ranging from three weeks to six months because of the symptoms, and 4 percent for more than six months. About 50 percent of the study population had at some time had symptoms related to the neck and 5 percent had been incapacitated from work because of their neck problems. In Hult's (44) survey of industrial and forest workers in Sweden, 80 percent reported having at some time had symptoms in the low back, and over half had been incapacitated by lumbago, lumbar insufficiency, or sciatica. About 80 percent said they had experienced symptoms in the neck region.

In the United States, data from the Health Interview Survey of the National Center for Health Statistics (77) show that impairments of the back and spine are the chronic conditions most frequently causing activity limitation among persons under 45 years of age, and that they rank third, after heart disease and the category arthritis and rheumatism, in persons of ages 45 to 64 years. A study from an Eastman Kodak plant in Rochester, New York (85), indicated that over a ten-year period, 45 percent of heavy handlers and 34 percent of sedentary workers visited the medical department for back pain. The majority of these workers were in their forties and fifties, so that there is a large impact of back pain among people in their productive years. That some of these workers will never return to productive employment was emphasized in a study of records from another industrial population (70).

Episodes of low back pain tend to start when people are in their twenties, and most of these attacks subside within one or two months. Recurrences are frequent, but tend to last for shorter periods of time than the initial episode. A Swedish study found that among people attributing their back problems to work injuries, lifting and twisting are the most frequently mentioned precipitating causes, while gardening is the most commonly mentioned leisure-time activity bringing about low back pain (76).

The vast majority of episodes of low back pain do not seriously incapacitate people. Of those seeking care for low back pain from family physicians, for instance, almost half improve in a week and almost 90 percent are better within a month, regardless of treatment (23). About 7 percent of people who have had episodes of back pain report that they still have the pain after six months; it is these patients who are primarily responsible for the high costs associated with low back injuries. Nachemson estimated that the relatively small proportion of chronic cases account for one-third of the costs, while Snook (90) has noted that among industrial workers, 25 percent of the cases account for 90 percent of the costs. Nachemson (76) found from a review of the literature that factors influencing the likelihood of recurrence include a first attack attributable to trauma, the presence of pain along the sciatic nerve, certain X-ray findings, alcoholism, psychosocial variables, and the size of associated insurance benefits. There is evidence that workers suffering industrial back injuries who report pain for more than three months are more likely to be disturbed emotionally than control patients (9).

Most studies concerned with risk factors for low back pain have been undertaken in industry, where the impact of low back pain is enormous. Snook (90) and Andersson (2,3) recently reviewed the epidemiology of low back pain in industry in detail, and much of the material presented will be from the information they have compiled. Note, however, that almost all the data are based on episodes of sickness-absence or on compensation claims; it is thus difficult to disentangle factors associated with the development of back pain from those related to ability to qualify for compensation or ability to perform a job once back pain has developed.

Snook (90) has found that although women and men are affected with low back pain with approximately equal frequency, work-related injuries for which compensation is received are much more common in men. The occupation with the highest rate of compensable back injuries is truck driving. Only 8 percent of the injuries occurred while driving trucks, and more than half were associated with loading and unloading the trucks. Material handlers have been found to be at next-highest risk for compensable back injuries, the injuries being associated with lifting, lowering, pushing, pulling, carrying, bending, twisting, falling, and slipping. High rates of compensable back injury are also present among nurses and nursing aides who have to perform many of the same types of tasks as those handling heavy objects in industry.

Andersson (2,3) reported six work-related factors to be associated with sickness-absence from low back pain, the first being the performance of physically heavy work. However, Andersson points out that the relative importance of various aspects of heavy work has not been clearly established and that workers in jobs requiring strenuous physical effort may lose time from work because they are unable to perform these strenuous jobs, whereas persons with less physically demanding jobs may not have to be absent from work. A second factor is work in the same position for long periods of time, including prolonged sitting, driving, or bent-over positions. A third frequently precipitating factor is lifting, although the evidence indicates that it is only jobs requiring very frequent heavy lifting that contribute to the development of symptoms. Sudden unexpected lifting may also be especially injurious. Fourth, bending and twisting, possibly in conjunction with lifting, are frequently associated with back injuries. Fifth, repetitive work, such as in assembly lines, is associated with a higher sickness-absence rate from low back pain as well as from other disorders. And, sixth, exposure to various types of vibration, such as in motor vehicles, increases the frequency of occurrence of back pain, possibly because repetitive small amounts of trauma can bring about permanent damage in the spine. Although industry has tried to prevent back injuries by careful selection of workers, training procedures, and job design, only good job design and perhaps strength testing (17) have been found to reduce substantially the frequency of compensable back injuries (90,91).

Other possible risk factors for low back pain not related to specific occupations include tallness (36), poor muscle strength (14), and smoking, presumably through the mechanism of frequent coughing (33,36). Body weight and posture have been considered as etiologic factors, but to date evidence on their role is conflicting. Although there is a general belief that psychological factors play a role in the etiology of low back pain, so far no studies have measured psychological variables before the onset of back pain. It is thus impossible to know whether certain psychological traits contribute to the development of the back pain or whether having back pain causes psychological disturbances such as depression, anxiety, fear, and excessive concern about one's health. In any event, there does not appear to be any one "pain personality" associated with low back pain patients (65,83).

In addition, although this discussion has focused on pain in the lower back, a large overlap exists among patients with shoulder, cervical spine, and lumbar spine disorders when complaint rates, abnormalities seen on X-ray, or conditions diagnosed clinically are considered, thus pointing out that the lumbar spine cannot be considered in isolation from other parts of the spine and the shoulders (96).

Finally, it must be reemphasized that in this discussion low back pain has been considered as a whole, and that the different lesions associated with low back pain undoubtedly have different etiologic characteristics. Prolonged sitting, for instance, may be associated with disc prolapses while lifting heavy materials may be related to sprains and strains of the muscles, ligaments, and other supporting structures. It is very important that future studies try to distinguish the different types of back pain. Prospective studies are needed in order to separate those factors leading to the development of back pain from those that occur as a consequence of back pain.

PROLAPSED INTERVERTEBRAL DISCS

In a prolapsed intervertebral disc (also known as a herniated disc, ruptured disc, or "slipped" disc), the gelatinous center of the disc, the nucleus pulposus, protrudes outside of its surrounding fibrocartilage ring, the annulus fibrosis. It most frequently protrudes in a posterior lateral direction, and when it does, the disc material tends to impinge on a nerve root (see Figure 6-1). In the low back the affected nerve runs down the leg, while in the neck, the affected nerve runs down the shoulder and arms. At the levels most frequently affected in the low back, this is the sciatic nerve. The usual symptoms of a prolapsed lumbar disc are pain in the low back and/or pain radiating down one or occasionally both legs along the course of the affected nerve, while in a prolapsed cervical disc, pain

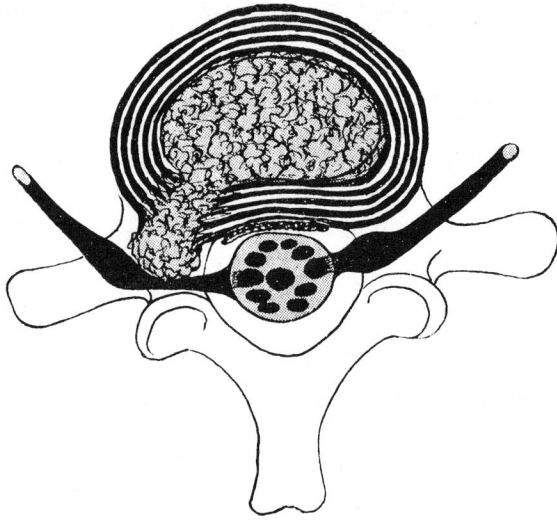

Figure 6-1   Prolapsed intervertebral disc, pressing on a nerve root.
Source: Aston (6).

usually occurs in the neck and/or radiates down an arm or occasionally both arms.

The U.S. Health Interview Survey (78) reports that each year more than one percent of persons in the age group 17 to 64 years state that they have trouble with a prolapsed intervertebral disc (called "a slipped or ruptured disc" in the checklist of diseases used in the Survey). The absence of diagnostic confirmation in these reports strongly suggests that this percentage is not really accurate, but it does give a general idea of the magnitude of the problem. Data from the U.S. Social Security Administration (95) show that among people under 40 years of age, prolapsed disc is second only to schizophrenia as the most frequent condition for which worker disability payments are allowed; if all ages are considered together, prolapsed disc is third, following chronic ischemic heart disease and osteoarthrosis. While the motive of secondary gain sometimes skews Social Security Administration statistics, this disorder clearly has a large impact on industrial populations.

Prolapsed Lumbar Intervertebral Discs

Prolapsed lumbar discs are seen considerably more frequently than prolapsed cervical discs. Using data from two studies of back pain seen by general practitioners in England (22,97), a survey of a general population in Copenhagen (36), and a study in an industrial population in England (34), a very rough estimate of the annual incidence of prolapsed lumbar intervertebral discs of around 0.1 to 0.5 percent per year in the population of ages 24 to 64 years may be made.

Lumbar disc prolapses are most often seen at the L-4 and L-5 levels (15,21,55,57,62,92,98), that is, in the disc between the fourth and fifth lumbar vertebrae and the disc between the fifth lumbar vertebra and the sacrum. For unknown reasons, prolapses at the L-4 level have been increasing in frequency relative to those at the L-5 level over the past few decades (92). Several reasons probably explain the predominance of prolapses at the L-4 and L-5 levels: (1) the posterior longitudinal ligament is narrower at the lower lumbar levels than the higher, thus providing less support for the discs; (2) most movement in the lumbar area takes place at these levels, thus subjecting these discs to more stress than those at higher levels; (3) the lumbar lordosis puts these discs at an angle further from the horizontal than those at higher levels, thereby making them more subject to stress from superincumbent weight than the discs at higher levels; and (4) torsion puts more pressure on the L-4 and L-5 discs than on higher discs (15,39). Males but not females are more likely to have pain radiating down their left leg than their right (52,55), indicating that disc protrusions occur more frequently to the left than to the right. The reasons for this are not known, however.

Most cases occur in individuals between 20 and 64 years of age. Cases undergoing surgery for lumbar disc prolapses are most frequently in the age group 30 to 39 years (1,24,40,42,52,80,98,106), although patients not undergoing surgery with similar symptoms are on the average somewhat younger than those who do undergo surgery (52). The exact explanation for the age distribution is not known, but the reduced frequency of prolapses in people older than 40 years of age is probably related to the loss of turgor and elasticity of discs with age, thus decreasing the likelihood of a prolapse occurring (43). At very young ages, the disc is well hydrated and resilient, making it mechanically less likely to fragment and prolapse. Thus, a disc may be at highest risk for prolapse while it is undergoing a change from a healthy resilient state with high water content to a relatively dry, scarred state (99).

Surgical case series generally indicate that prolapsed lumbar discs are more common in males than in females. Spangfort (92), for example, reported a ratio of males to females of 2 to 1 in 52 published case series. On the other hand, no excess of male patients has been observed among individuals with similar signs and symptoms who do not have surgery (37,42,52). The results of one study (52) and clinical impression suggest that for the same degree of symptomatology, men are more likely to have surgery than women; therefore, the excess of males among surgical patients may be at least partially attributable to their greater likelihood of surgery. The actual male-to-female ratio is not known, and in fact probably cannot be determined.

Several studies (35,41,51) suggest that the driving of motor vehicles increases the risk for prolapsed lumbar discs. Both occupational driving, including truck and bus driving, and other types of driving appear to be involved. It is not known exactly which aspects of driving are responsible for the increased risk, but several factors could be involved. For instance, the vibratory forces imposed upon the spine during driving may be a causative mechanism (35). Sudden starting and stopping has also been postulated as a source of mechanical stress (5). From a model of the human spine, Arvikar and Seireg (5) found that sudden forward acceleration resulted in high cervical disc pressures while sudden backward acceleration resulted in high lumbar disc pressures. Other possible reasons are the lack of proper support for the back in many motor vehicles, and the position of the driver's legs, which may put stress on the spine since the legs are extended to the floor pedals rather than flat on the floor. A driver's inability to alter his or her position to any great extent may play a role as well. Modes of transportation other than motor vehicles need to be studied; passengers in airplanes, for instance, are also exposed to vibration and to prolonged sitting in one position.

Individuals who have had sedentary occupations for several years may also have an elevated risk for prolapsed lumbar disc (49). This finding needs to be confirmed in other studies, but it is consistent with the experimental evidence that there is more pressure on the discs in a sitting position than when a person is standing or lying down (15,47,75). An association of sedentary occupations with prolapsed lumbar discs could also explain why some studies (36,67), which have focused on the epidemiology of low back pain in general rather than on specific disease entities, have noted an association of low back pain with both very sedentary and very physically demanding occupations. Prolapsed discs may be related to sedentary occupations while such conditions as muscle strains and injuries to the ligaments are associated with heavy occupations. Jobs involving lifting, pushing, pulling, and carrying have been reported not to be associated with prolapsed lumbar discs (49), but, again, further study is needed. Although an activity such as lifting is sometimes reported to have precipitated the onset of symptoms, it may not have much importance as an underlying etiologic factor. Of relevance to this, it has been found that lumbar discs are very resistant to compression loads; from experiments performed on autopsy specimens it has been learned that compression loads will fracture vertebral end plates before they damage discs (28).

Epidemiologic studies have so far not considered risks associated with jobs involving frequent twisting. Since experimental and theoretical evidence indicates that torsion may cause pathologic changes in the intervertebral discs (26–28,39), it is important that epidemiologic studies examine this question. Occupations requiring frequent bending should also be considered (39).

One study reported that full-term pregnancies increase the risk for prolapsed lumbar discs at the L-5 level (50). This is biologically plausible, since both mechanical stress from carrying and delivering the baby and ligamentous laxity toward the end of pregnancy produced by the hormone relaxin from the corpus luteum could elevate the risk.

A study in a military population indicated that men with defects of the back and legs at the time of induction were more likely than other men to have subsequent prolapsed discs (41). However, it is possible that these defects were actually early manifestations of the disease, so that it is not known whether the defects were of etiologic significance. Tallness has also been found to be associated with an increased risk for low back pain with sciatica (41,48,59).

Other risk factors for prolapsed lumbar discs have been suggested in individual studies, including chronic cough and chronic bronchitis (36,48), insufficient physical activity (48), participation in baseball, golf, and bowling (48), the spring and fall seasons (44,48), posture (41), and a heavy body frame (41). Possible biological mechanisms for some of these risk factors could be suggested. Frequent coughing, for example, would put more pressure on the discs; insufficient physical activity would adversely affect muscle tone; the swinging motions in baseball and golf involve torsion; and posture and body build could affect the amount of stress on the disc.

Physical trauma was formerly believed to be *the* cause of prolapsed discs (19), but since many prolapsed discs occur without any antecedent trauma and since most people do suffer trauma to their backs from time to time, other factors must be involved. Today, trauma is seldom regarded as *the* underlying cause, although it is sometimes the precipitating event (20,48,68).

Psychological factors in low back pain have been considered in some studies, but only a few investigations have focused specifically on prolapsed discs. Scott (89) presented his clinical impression that emotional stress is related to prolapsed discs, and found in experiments with voles that the fluid content of their discs changed when the voles were subjected to emotional stress. It has been hypothesized (63) that an increase in intracellular sodium in depressed patients could cause discs to swell and become more susceptible to prolapses. Neither of these findings has been confirmed or refuted in human epidemiologic studies. Nevertheless, prolonged stress apparently does result in contraction of back muscles (15,88), which in turn increases pressure on the discs, thereby decreasing their ability to absorb fluids (15). The etiologic role of emotional stress merits further investigation, if the appropriate study design could be devised.

Heredity is also often postulated to be a possible etiologic factor in prolapsed discs (20). A proper study of the role of heredity would involve thorough and extensive study of prolapsed discs in families, with similar diagnostic criteria applied to case and control family members.

Prolapsed Cervical Intervertebral Discs

No epidemiologic studies of prolapsed cervical discs have apparently been published. In a neurosurgical practice it was observed that the ratio of prolapsed cervical discs to lumbar discs seen at surgery was 1 to 10 in 1966 (72), but 1 to 8 in 1973 (73,74). Whether these data represent a true change in the relative frequency of lesions in these two areas over time or merely reflect changes in referral, diagnostic, or treatment patterns is not known.

Cervical disc prolapses tend to occur in a slightly older age group than do lumbar disc prolapses. Hult (44), for instance, found that brachialgia (pain in the arm or arms) occurs most frequently in the 35 to 49 year old age group, and surgical case series (69,107) indicate that individuals in the age group 40 to 49 years are the ones most likely to have surgery for prolapsed cervical discs. Little difference has been reported between females and males in the proportion affected with brachialgia (60), but surgical case series (69,107), which are undoubtedly not representative of the general population, indicate a male predominance for cervical prolapsed discs. The true sex ratio is not known.

Prolapses are most frequently seen at surgery at the C-6 and C-5 levels (69,73,74,107). Like the L-4 and L-5 discs in the lumbar spine, the C-6 and C-5 discs are subject to more stress than are other cervical discs.

The majority of patients treated for cervical disc prolapses do not report a history of injury preceding the onset of symptoms (107). An etiologic role for heavy physical activity is perhaps unlikely, since brachialgia has been reported with about equal frequency by forest and industrial workers (44), and by men doing heavy and light work (43). The men doing heavy work were found to be more incapacitated by their brachialgia than those doing light work (44), but this sheds no light on etiology. Prolonged stress in the neck area could be involved, however, since workers in the food industry were at excess risk for brachialgia in one of the Swedish studies (44), a finding that might be attributable to the tendency of these workers to carry heavy carcasses on their shoulders. Attention should also be paid to jobs requiring a lot of twisting of the neck because of the experimental and theoretical evidence that torsion is damaging to discs (26–28,39).

Other than these few observations, little has been reported on the characteristics of people who develop prolapsed cervical intervertebral discs. Also, the extent to which risk factors are similar for lumbar and cervical prolapsed discs is not known. It seems likely that some factors such as driving might affect discs in both the cervical and lumbar regions whereas other sources of stress would be specific for either the neck or low back. Even basic demographic characteristics of surgical and nonsurgical cases such as age, sex, and ethnic group need to be determined, since they are of interest in their own right and may provide leads to additional etiologic agents.

DISC DEGENERATION

Degenerated intervertebral discs have lost their fluid and elasticity, and are rather dry and scarred. As discs degenerate, the space between the vertebrae usually narrows, and as this narrowing progresses, marginal osteophytosis (bony outgrowths) of the vertebrae may occur. To a large extent, disc degeneration may be considered as part of the normal aging process, and many people with X-ray evidence of disc degeneration have no symptoms. Why some people with disc degeneration have symptoms while many do not is not at all clear (45,87). Pain in the cervical area has been found to be associated with positive X-ray findings only in individuals younger than 45 years of age, while pain in the lumbar region was associated with X-ray changes only in individuals under 54 years of age (61). Others (43,44) have found very little association between disc degeneration and symptomatology unless there are other changes secondary to the disc degeneration. Results have also been somewhat conflicting as to how frequently nerve root impingement results from the foraminal narrowing that often occurs with disc degeneration (45,60,81,87). The clinical significance and consequences of disc degeneration are thus unclear.

Population studies indicate that disc degeneration is indeed common, but their meaning is difficult to interpret since they are cross-sectional and rely on narrowing of the disc space as an indicator of disc degeneration. It is well recognized that disc spaces may be narrowed either because of a disc prolapse or from the desiccation and degeneration of discs; narrowing from either of these sources may lead to osteophytosis of the vertebral rims (11). Although in young adults a certain amount of disc degeneration may be associated with disc prolapses, once the degeneration has reached an advanced state, the likelihood of a prolapse is substantially decreased (4,18). Therefore, one should distinguish degenerated discs from prolapsed discs in epidemiologic studies.

In a study of persons in the age range 55 to 64 years in a town in northern England (53), disc degeneration, as indicated by narrowing of the disc space and osteophytosis, was observed in about 70 percent of the lumbar spines and cervical spines of men, and in about 60 percent of the cervical spines and 50 percent of the lumbar spines of women. It has generally been found that disc degeneration is more common in males than in females, particularly in the severe forms of the disease (59–61). Prevalence rates for disc degeneration increase steeply with age in both the cervical and lumbar regions (30,31,44,60). In one general population study (see Figure 6-2) (60) cervical disc degeneration graded as minimal, moderate, or severe (grades 2 to 4) was found in the X-rays of less than 1 percent of males in the age group 15 to 24 years but in 88 percent of those 65 to 74 years of age. Moderate or severe degeneration in the lumbar area was noted in 36 percent of those in the age group 35 to 44 and in 85 percent of those aged 65 to 74 years. Even in people who have been completely asymptomatic, Figure 6-3 shows that the prevalence of degenerative changes in the cervical discs increases markedly with age (31). Autopsy studies indicate that disc degeneration begins in the 20 to 25 year group and usually progresses to marginal osteophytosis only after the age of 45 years (64). The levels most frequently affected are those subject to the most stress: the L5-S1 and L4-L5 levels in the lumbar spine and the C5-C6, C6-C7, and C4-C5 levels in the cervical spine (15,31,81,82).

Although degenerated discs occur in both the cervical and lumbar spines of the same individuals more often than would be anticipated by

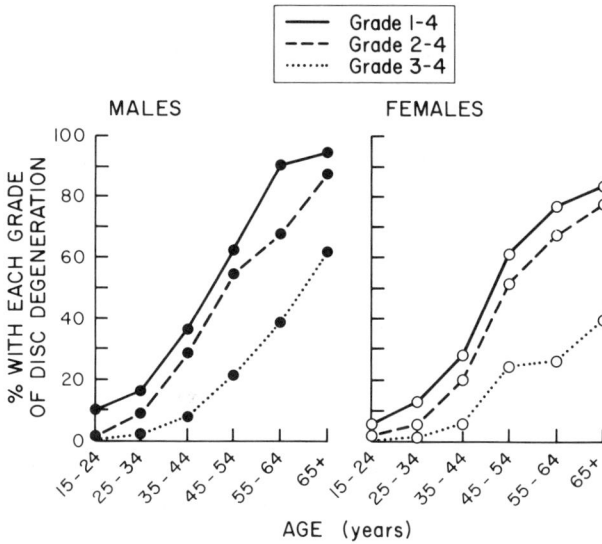

Figure 6-2 Prevalence rate of cervical disc degeneration, by grade of degeneration, in population surveys in the United Kingdom.

Source: Lawrence (60).

Figure 6-3 Ratio of asymptomatic individuals with and without degeneration of a cervical intervertebral disc, by age. Equal numbers of men and women are included in each group.

Source: Friedenberg and Miller (31).

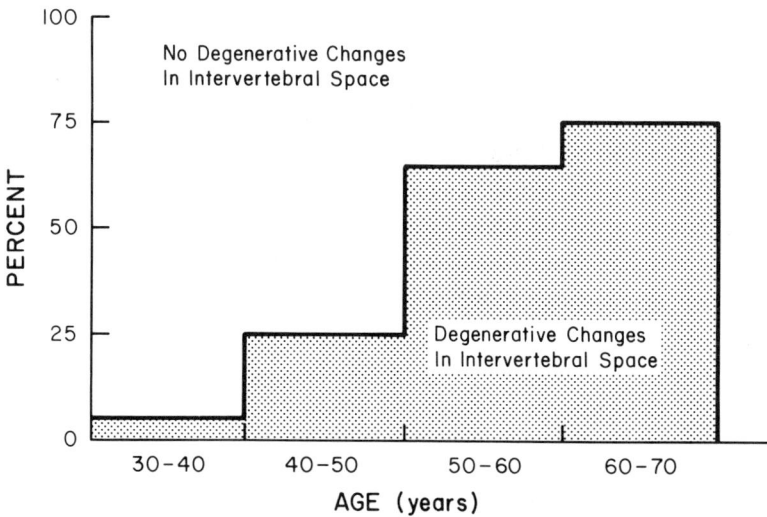

chance (12,60), there is no evidence of a specific constitutional factor except in rare instances. Disc degeneration does not seem to be related to generalized osteoarthrosis (54). Mechanical stress to the spine is associated with the development of degenerative disc disease in the lumbar spine (16,53,54,59,60), but the nature of the stress is uncertain. Among the occupations with high prevalence rates of degenerative disc disease are miners (16,59,60), dock workers (59), and outdoor workers such as farmers and road builders (60), but there is disagreement as to whether stress from heavy lifting or from injuries and repeated trauma is the reason for this high prevalence (16,59). One group of investigators (61) has reported that degenerative disc disease is rare in the lumbar spines of sedentary workers. Obesity does not appear to be a risk factor for degenerative disc disease (60).

Occupational stress from heavy jobs, however, does not seem to be an important etiologic factor for degenerative cervical disc disease (12,53,60), although very severe degeneration has been noted in coal miners and unskilled laborers (60). One study (11) suggested that while occupational stress may not be involved in the initiation of the degenerative process, it may increase risk for neurologic complications once degeneration exists. Cervical disc degeneration has been found to be more common in Jamaica than in England; this might be attributed to the tendency of Jamaicans to carry heavy loads on their heads (13). Thus, further studies are needed that specifically consider stress on the neck.

Finally, an autoimmune mechanism has been suggested as being etiologically involved (10). Since the mucoprotein in the nucleus pulposus of the disc is avascular, this protein or one or more of its degradation products could become involved in an autoimmune reaction if it were exposed to circulating blood.

In summary, more is known about risk factors for lumbar than for cervical degenerative disc disease. In both parts of the spine, however, age is the best predictor of degenerative disc disease. This makes it difficult to determine to what extent disc degeneration is due to exogenous factors and to what extent it is an inevitable consequence of aging. Mechanical stress is important too, but much remains to be learned about the nature of the mechanical stress that hastens the degenerative process.

SPONDYLOLISTHESIS

Spondylolisthesis consists of gradual forward displacement of one vertebra over the one beneath. This displacement usually occurs because of

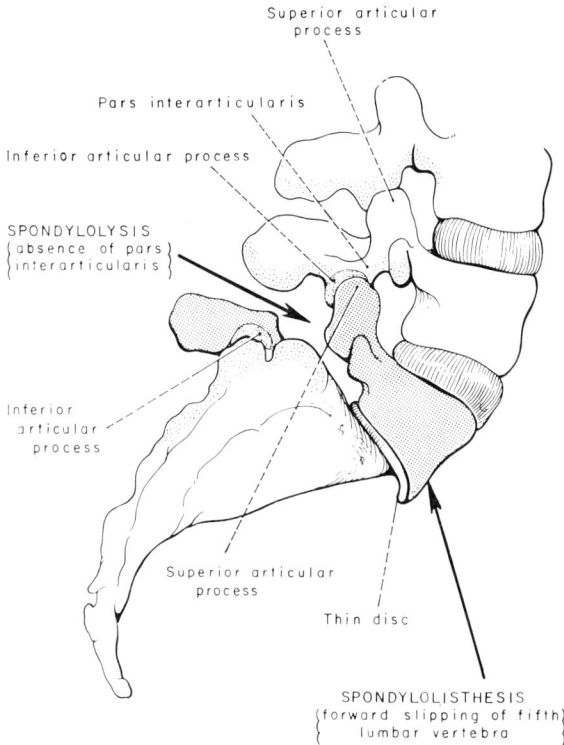

Figure 6-4 Spondylolisthesis and spondylolysis.

Source: MacAusland and Mayo (66).

the presence of spondylolysis, a defect in the pars interarticularis of the neural arch (see Figure 6-4). Occasionally, trauma to areas other than the pars interarticularis permits the displacement. Many affected individuals are asymptomatic and spondylolisthesis is diagnosed in them only if it is seen incidently on X-ray. Other persons have low back pain which, if there is nerve root compression, may radiate into one or both legs. Weakness and stiffness of the spinal column are also common. The L-5 level is most frequently affected, followed by L-4, L-3, L-2, and L-1, respectively (32). Spondylolysis and spondylolisthesis are not known to occur in animals other than man, suggesting that upright posture may predispose to this condition (101). These disorders do not occur in the ape or other primates (101).

Prevalence rates of spondylolysis in adults in Western countries are around 5 percent, as determined from X-ray findings and from skeletons.

About half of these individuals have developed spondylolisthesis, with the extent of displacement usually not more than 25 to 30 percent (7,8,84,86,100). Much higher prevalence rates have been found in skeletons of Alaskan Eskimos and Aleuts north of the Yukon River (93).

X-ray studies and surveys of skeletons have shown an enormous increase in pars interarticularis defects between the ages of 5.5 and 6.5 years, although in most children symptoms are not apparent at this time. The prevalence of these defects increases slightly through the adolescent years, with very little further increase during the adult years (8,84,104). The increase in prevalence around 6 years of age has been hypothesized to occur because children start to push and shove each other around at school or because for the first time they sit for long periods of time with a lordotic posture (102).

It is not clear why some individuals with spondylolysis develop spondylolisthesis while others do not, although it is likely that physical stress on the spine is involved (46). The slippage is probably a gradual process, starting shortly after age 6 to 7 years and for some reason accelerating between the ages of 9 and 17 years. If displacement occurs, it will generally happen before 18 years of age; displacement rarely takes place at older ages (58,102). Symptoms often do not occur immediately following displacement, and one report (32) indicates that spondylolisthesis is most frequently *diagnosed* among males of ages 31 to 40 years and among females of ages 41 to 50 years.

In the United States, whites are affected more frequently with spondylolysis and spondylolisthesis than blacks and males more often than females (84,104). However, a recent study from South Africa (25) found similar prevalence rates for spondylolysis in blacks and whites and in males and females; the reasons for these discrepant results are unknown.

Spondylolysis and spondylolisthesis occur much more frequently than would be expected by chance in association with spina bifida at the L-5 level (25,46,84,105). It has been suggested that if spina bifida is present there is less support from ligaments and a greater amount of pivotal strain across the pars interarticularis of the affected vertebra during extension (25). Spondylolisthesis is probably also associated with lumbosacral segmental defects (84,105).

Familial aggregation of spondylolysis and spondylolisthesis cases is marked (7,8,32,38,100,105), strongly suggesting a hereditary predisposition with an as-yet-unknown mode of inheritance. Results from one study (105) indicate no association with length of gestation, type of presentation, birth weight, season of birth, social class, or a previous maternal miscarriage or stillbirth.

The relationship of physical activity to the development of spondylolysis and spondylolisthesis has received much attention. Gymnasts, American football players, persons practicing karate, and others with a high degree of stress in their lumbar spine have been reported to be at high risk for pars articularis defects and subsequent spondylolisthesis (46). Although it has been hypothesized that overweight individuals have a greater likelihood of spondylolysis (71), apparently no data exist to support or refute this. Stewart (93) suggested that unusual postural stress, a high accident rate, and possibly a high frequency of anomalous ossification could contribute to the high prevalence of neural arch defects in northern Alaskan skeletons.

Biomechanics specialists have suggested that specific motions during physical activity could contribute to neural arch defects and to displacement. Three mechanisms could act separately or in combination to cause failure of the neural arch, with or without displacement of the vertebral body: flexion overload, unbalanced stress forces, and forced rotation (29). Torsion was found to be the most detrimental of these forces. Since the antitorsional forces of a child are less well developed than those in an adult, this could explain the young age at onset. Both Farfan et al. (29) and Kraus (56) suggest that flatter spines are more likely to fail by flexion and spines with more lordosis to fail from torsion. Troup (94), on the other hand, feels that extension of the spine could be an important contributing factor to spondylolisthesis when consideration is given to the roles of the supporting muscles, the stiffness of the intervertebral disc, as well as to the motion involved in extension. Thus, the specific motions that contribute to the likelihood of displacement are not yet established.

Much confusion and contradiction has existed about the etiology of spondylolisthesis, part of which may have resulted from failure to consider separately several etiologically distinct types of spondylolisthesis. Wiltse, Newman, and Macnab (103) have proposed the following five etiologic categories of spondylolisthesis to account for various observations on the roles of heredity and environmental factors:

1. Dysplastic spondylolisthesis, which results from congenital dysplasia of the upper sacrum on the neural arch of L-5. Because there is insufficient strength to withstand the forward thrust of superincumbent body weight, the last free vertebra gradually slips forward on the one below and the pars interarticularis usually either elongates or breaks apart. No accurate statistics are available on its frequency, but it occurs at an early age and is twice as common in girls as in boys.

2. Isthmic spondylolisthesis, which is the most common type and which results from a lesion in the pars interarticularis; it may be divided into

three subtypes. Subtype A (lytic), in which there is a strong hereditary component, consists of separation or dissolution of the pars, and a fatigue fracture is always present. A marked increase in frequency occurs between the ages of 5.5 and 6.5 years and some increase between 11 and 15 years of age, the latter possibly because very strenuous athletic activities lead to fatigue fractures. It is not known whether the fracture in the pars results from flexion or extension stresses. Subtype B (elongation of the pars without separation) also occurs secondarily to fatigue microfractures and shows familial aggregation. Subtype C (acute pars fracture) is always secondary to severe trauma, and heredity is probably not important.

3. Degenerative spondylolisthesis, which results from long-standing intersegmental instability and which occurs six to nine times more frequently at the L-4 level than at either the L-3 or L-5 level. Slipping is usually less than 30 percent. The predisposing factor is thought to be a straight, stable lumbosacral joint that places increased stress on the intervertebral joint between the fourth and fifth lumbar vertebrae; this leads to decompression of the ligaments, hypermobility, and degeneration of the articular processes, thus allowing forward slipping. This is never seen below the age of 40 and seldom below the age of 50 years. It occurs about four times more frequently among women than men and three times more frequently among blacks than whites. It occurs four times more frequently when the fifth lumbar vertebra is sacralized than when it is not.

4. Traumatic spondylolisthesis, which only occurs secondarily to a severe acute injury that fractures some part of the posterior element other than the pars and allows forward slip of the vertebra above on the one below.

5. Pathologic spondylolisthesis, which results from local or generalized bone disease in the posterior element mechanism. The underlying disease weakens the mechanism so that it cannot hold against the forward thrust of superincumbent body weight, and a vertebra slips forward on the one below.

Newman and Stone (79) have found that traumatic and pathologic spondylolisthesis are rare, while spondylotic spondylolisthesis is the most frequent, and congenital and degenerative spondylolisthesis occur with intermediate frequency. This relative frequency is consistent with the observed age distribution of spondylolisthesis.

Further data are needed to evaluate this classification scheme. Wynne-Davies and Scott (105) have found that relatives of patients affected with either the dysplastic or isthmic forms are at higher risks for either of these specific forms than are individuals from the general population, indicating that additional studies are needed of the extent to which a positive family history of one form predisposes to another form.

REFERENCES

1. Aitken, A. P. 1952. "Rupture of the intervertebral disc." *Amer. J. Surg.* 84:261–267.
2. Andersson, G. B. J. 1979. "Low back pain in industry: Epidemiological aspects." *Scand. J. Rehab. Med.* 11:163–168.
3. ———. 1981. "Epidemiological aspects on low back pain in industry." *Spine.* G:53–60, 1981.
4. Anonymous. 1958. "Physical changes in the prolapsed disc." *Lancet* 2:1214–1215.
5. Arvikar, R. J., and Seireg, A. 1978. "Distribution of spinal disc pressures in the seated posture subjected to impact." *Aviat., Space, and Environ. Med.* 49:166–169.
6. Aston, J. N. 1967. *A Short Textbook of Orthopaedics and Traumatology.* Philadelphia: Lippincott.
7. Bailey, W. 1947. "Observations on the etiology and frequency of spondylolisthesis and its precursors." *Radiology* 48:107–113.
8. Baker, D. R., and McHollic, W. 1956. "Spondyloschisis and spondylolisthesis in children." Proc. Amer. Acad. Orthop. Surg. *J. Bone Jt. Surg. (Amer.)* 38:933–934.
9. Beals, R. K., and Hickman, N. W. 1972. "Industrial injuries of the back and extremities." *J. Bone Jt. Surg. (Amer.)* 54:1593–1611.
10. Bobechko, W. P., and Hirsch, C. 1965. "Auto-immune response to nucleus pulposus in the rabbit." *J. Bone Jt. Surg. (Brit.)* 47:574–580.
11. Bradshaw, P. 1957. "Some aspects of cervical spondylosis." *Quart. J. Med.* 26:177–208.
12. Brain, W. R. 1954. "Spondylosis, the known and the unknown." *Lancet* 1:687–693.
13. Bremner, J., Lawrence, J. S., and Miall, W. E. 1968. "Degenerative joint disease in a Jamaican rural population." *Ann. Rheum. Dis.* 27:326–332.
14. Cady, L. D., Bischoff, D. P., O'Connell, E. R., Thomas, P. C., and Allen, J. H. 1979. "Strength and fitness and subsequent back injuries in firefighters." *J. Occup. Med.* 21:269–272.
15. Caillet, R. 1968. *Low Back Pain Syndrome.* Philadelphia: F. A. Davis Company.
16. Caplan, P. S., Freedman, L. M. J., and Connelly, T. P. 1966. "Degenerative joint disease of the lumbar spine in coal miners—a clinical and x-ray study." *Arthritis Rheum.* 9:693–702.
17. Chaffin, D. B., Herrin, G. D., and Keyserling, W. M. 1978. "Preemployment strength testing. An updated position." *J. Occup. Med.* 20:403–408.
18. Charnley, J. 1952. "The imbibition of fluid as a cause of herniation of the nucleus pulposus." *Lancet* 1:124–127.
19. Coventry, M. B., Ghormley, R. K., and Kernohan, J. W. 1945. "The intervertebral disc: Its microscopic anatomy and pathology. Part III, Pathologic changes in the intervertebral disc." *J. Bone Jt. Surg.* 27:460–474.

20. ———. 1968. "Low back and sciatic pain. Introduction to symposium." *J. Bone Jt. Surg. (Amer.)* 50:167–169.
21. DePalma, A. F., and Rothman, R. H. 1970. *The Intervertebral Disc.* Philadelphia: Saunders.
22. Dillane, J. B., Fry, J., and Kalton, G. 1966. "Acute back syndrome—A study from general practice." *Brit. Med. J.* 2:82–84.
23. Dixon, A. St. J. 1973. "Progress and problems in back pain research." *Rheum. Rehab.* 12:165–174.
24. Eckert, C., and Decker, A. 1947. "Pathological studies of intervertebral discs." *J. Bone Jt. Surg. (Amer.)* 29:447–460.
25. Eisenstein, S. 1978. "A skeletal investigation of two population groups." *J. Bone Jt. Surg. (Brit.)* 60:488–494.
26. Farfan, H. F. 1969. "Effects of torsion on the intervertebral joints." *Can. J. Surg.* 12:336–341.
27. ———, Cossette, J. W., Robertson, G. H., Wells, R. W., and Kraus, H. 1970. "The effects of torsion on the lumbar intervertebral joints: The role of torsion in the production of disc degeneration." *J. Bone Jt. Surg. (Amer.)* 52:468–497.
28. ———, Huberdeau, R. M., and Dubow, H. I. 1972. "Lumbar intervertebral disc degeneration." *J. Bone Jt. Surg. (Amer.)* 54:492–510.
29. ———, Osterin, V., and Lamy, C. 1976. "The mechanical etiology of spondylolysis and spondylolisthesis." *Clin. Orthop.* 117:40–55.
30. Friedenberg, Z. B., Edeiken, J., Spencer, H. N., and Tolentino, S. C. 1959. "Degenerative changes in the cervical spine." *J. Bone Jt. Surg. (Amer.)* 41:61–70.
31. ———, and Miller, W. T. 1963. "Degenerative disc disease of the cervical spine." *J. Bone Jt. Surg. (Amer.)* 45:1171–1178.
32. Friberg, S. 1939. "Studies on spondylolisthesis." *Acta Chir. Scand. Suppl.* 55:1–140.
33. Frymoyer, J. W., Pope, M. H., Costanza, M. C., Rosen, J. C., Goggin, J. E., and Wilder, D. G. 1980. "Epidemiologic studies of low-back pain." *Spine* 5:419–423.
34. Glover, J. R. 1970. "Occupational health research and the problem of back pain." *Trans. Soc. Occup. Med.* 21:2–12.
35. Gruber, G. J., and Ziperman, H. H. 1974. *Relationship Between Whole-Body Vibration and Morbidity Patterns Among Motor Coach Operators.* Washington, D.C.,: HEW Publication No. (NIOSH) 75–104.
36. Gyntelberg, F. 1974. "One year incidence of low back pain among male residents of Copenhagen aged 40–59." *Dan. Med. Bull.* 21:30–36.
37. Hanraets, P. R. M. 1959. *The Degenerative Back.* Amsterdam: Elsevier.
38. Haukipuro, L., Keranen, N., Koivisto, E., Lindholm, R., Norio, R., and Punto, L. 1978. "Familial occurrence of lumbar spondylolysis and spondylolisthesis." *Clin. Genet.* 13:471–476.
39. Hickey, D. S., and Hukins, D. W. L. 1980. "Relation between the structure of the annulus fibrosus and the function of the intervertebral disc." *Spine* 5:106–116.
40. Hirsch, C., and Nachemson, A. 1963. "The reliability of lumbar disc surgery." *Clin. Orthop.* 29:189–195.
41. Hrubec, A., and Nashbold, B. S., Jr. 1975. "Epidemiology of lumbar disc lesions in the military in World War II." *Amer. J. Epidemiol.* 102:366–376.
42. Hudgins, W. R. 1970. "The predictive value of myelography in the diagnosis of ruptured lumbar discs." *J. Neurosurg.* 32:152–162.
43. Hult, L. 1954. "Cervical, dorsal, and lumbar spinal syndromes." *Acta Orthop. Scand. Suppl.* 17:1–102.

44. ——— 1954. "The Munkfors Investigation." *Acta Orthop. Scand. Suppl.* 16:1–76.
45. Hussar, A. E., and Guller, E. J. 1956. "Correlation of pain and the roentgenographic findings of spondylosis of the cervical and lumbar spine." *Amer. J. Med. Sci.* 232:518–527.
46. Jackson, D. W., Wiltse, L. L., and Cirincioni, R. J. 1976. "Spondylolysis in the female gymnast." *Clin. Orthop.* 117:68–73.
47. Keegan, J. 1953. "Alterations of the lumbar curve related to posture and seating." *J. Bone Jt. Surg. (Amer.)* 35:589–603.
48. Kelsey, J. L. 1975. "An epidemiological study of acute herniated lumbar intervertebral discs." *Rheumatol. Rehabil.* 14:144–155.
49. ———. 1975. "An epidemiological study of the relationship between occupations and acute herniated lumbar discs." *Int. J. Epid.* 4:197–205.
50. ———, Greenberg, R. A., Hardy, R. J., and Johnson, M. F. 1975. "Pregnancy and the syndrome of herniated lumbar intervertebral disc, an epidemiological study." *Yale J. Biol. Med.,* 48:361–368.
51. ———, and Hardy, R. J. 1975. "Driving of motor vehicles as a risk factor for acute herniated lumbar intervertebral disc." *Amer. J. Epid.* 102:63–73.
52. ———, and Ostfeld, A. M. 1975. "Demographic characteristics of persons with acute herniated lumbar intervertebral disc." *J. Chronic Dis.* 28:37–50.
53. Kellgren, J. H. 1961. "Osteoarthrosis in patients and populations." *Brit. Med. J.* 2:1–6.
54. ———, and Lawrence, J. S. 1958. "Osteo-arthrosis and disk degeneration in an urban population." *Ann. Rheum. Dis.* 17:388–396.
55. Knutsson, B. 1961. "Comparative value of electromyographic, myelographic and clinical-neurological examinations in diagnosis of lumbar nerve root compression." *Acta Orthop. Scand. Suppl.* 49:1–135.
56. Kraus, H. 1976. "Effect of lordosis on the stress in the lumbar spine." *Clin. Orthop.* 117:56–58.
57. Lansche, W. E., and Ford, L. T. 1960. "Correlation of the myelogram with clinical and operative findings in lumbar disc lesions." *J. Bone Jt. Surg. (Amer.)* 42:173–201.
58. Laurent, L. E., and Einola, S. 1961. "Spondylolischisis in children and adolescents." *Acta Orthop. Scand.* 31:45–64.
59. Lawrence, J. S. 1955. "Rheumatism in coal miners, part III: Occupational factors." *Brit. J. Ind. Med.* 12:249–261.
60. ———. 1969. "Disc degeneration, its frequency and relationship to symptoms." *Ann. Rheum. Dis.* 28:121–137.
61. ———, Degraaff, R., and Laine, V. A. J. 1963. "Degenerative joint disease in random samples and occupational groups." In *The Epidemiology of Chronic Rheumatism.* Vol. 1. J. H. Kellgren, ed. Oxford: Blackwell, pp. 98–119.
62. Lenhard, R. W. 1947. "End-result study of the intervertebral disc." *J. Bone Jt. Surg. (Amer.)* 29:425–428.
63. Levine, M. E. 1971. "Depression, back pain, and disc protrusion." *Dis. Nerv. Sys.* 32:41–45.
64. Levin, T. 1964. "Osteoarthritis in lumbar synovial joints, a morphologic study." *Acta Orthop. Scand. Suppl.* 73:1–112.
65. Louks, J. L., Freeman, C. W., and Calsyn, D. A. 1978. "Personality organization and back pain." *J. Person. Assess.* 42:152–158.
66. MacAusland, W. R., Jr., and Mayo, R. A. 1965. *Orthopedics.* Boston: Little Brown.
67. Magora, A. 1974. "Investigation of the relation between low back pain and occupation. Six medical histories and symptoms." *Scand. J. Rehabil. Med.* 6:81–88.

68. Martin, G. 1978. "The role of trauma in disc protrusion." *New Zeal. Med. J.* 87:208–211.
69. Martin, G. M., and Corbin, K. B. 1954. "An evaluation of conservative treatment for patients with cervical disk syndrome." *Arch. Phys. Med. Rehabil.* 35:87–91.
70. McGill, C. M. 1968. "Industrial back problems, a control program." *J. Occup. Med.* 10:174–178.
71. Monticelli, G., and Ascani, E. 1975. "Spondylolysis and spondylolisthesis." *Acta Orthop. Scand.* 46:498–506.
72. Murphey, F., and Simmons, J. C. H. 1966. "Ruptured cervical disc. Experience with 250 cases." *Amer. Surg.* 32:83–88.
73. ———, Simmons J. C. H., and Brunson, B. 1973. "Ruptured cervical discs, 1939 to 1972." *Clin. Neurosurg.* 20:9–17.
74. ——— et al. 1973. "Surgical treatment of laterally ruptured cervical disc. Review of 648 cases, 1939 to 1972." *J. Neurosurg.* 38:679–683.
75. Nachemson, A. 1965. "*In vivo* discometry in lumbar discs with irregular radiograms." *Acta Orthop. Scand.* 36:418–434.
76. ———. 1982. "The natural course of low back pain." In *Workshop on Idiopathic Low Back Pain.* St. Louis: The C. V. Mosby Co. In press.
77. National Center for Health Statistics. 1973. *Limitation of Activity Due to Chronic Conditions, United States, 1969–1970.* Series 10, Number 80.
78. National Center for Health Statistics. 1974. *Chronic Conditions Causing Activity Limitation, United States, 1969–1970.* Series 10, Number 96.
79. Newman, P. H., and Stone, K. H. 1963. "The etiology of spondylolisthesis." *J. Bone Jt. Surg. (Brit.)* 45:39–59.
80. O'Connell, J. E. A. 1960. "Lumbar disc protrusions in pregnancy." *J. Neurol. Neurosurg. Psych.* 23:138–141.
81. Palles, C., Jones, A. M., and Spillane, J. D. 1954. "Cervical spondylosis, incidence and implications." *Brain* 77:274–289.
82. Payne, E. E., and Spillane, J. D. 1957. "The cervical spine, an anatomico-pathological study of 70 specimens (using a special technique) with particular reference to the problem of cervical spondylosis." *Brain* 80:571–596.
83. Poussaint, A. F. 1982. "Psychological/psychiatric factors in the low back pain patient." In *Workshop on Idiopathic Low Back Pain.* St. Louis: The C. V. Mosby Co. In press.
84. Roche, M. B., and Rowe, G. G. 1952. "The incidence of separate neural arch and coincident bone variations. A summary." *J. Bone Jt. Surg. (Amer.)* 34:491–494.
85. Rowe, M. L. 1969. "Low back pain in industry. A position paper." *J. Occup. Med.* 11:161–169.
86. ———. 1971. "Low back disability in industry; updated position." *J. Occup. Med.* 13:476–478.
87. Rothman, R. H. 1973. "The pathophysiology of disc degeneration." *Clin. Neurosurg.* 20:174–182.
88. Sainsbury, P., and Gibson, J. G. 1954. "Symptoms of anxiety and tension and the accompanying physiological changes in muscular system." *J. Neurol. Neurosurg. Psych.* 17:216–224.
89. Scott, J. C. 1955. "Stress factor in disc syndrome." *J. Bone Jt. Surg. (Brit.)* 37:107–111.
90. Snook, S. H. 1982. "Low back pain in industry." In *Workshop on Idiopathic Low Back Pain.* St. Louis: The C. V. Mosby Co. In press.
91. ———, Campanelli, R. A., and Hart, J. W. 1978. "A study of three preventive approaches to low back injury." *J. Occup. Med.* 20:478–481.
92. Spangfort, E. V. 1972. "The lumbar disc herniation, a computer-aided analysis of 2504 operations." *Acta Orthop. Scand. Supp.* 142:1–95.

93. Stewart, T. D. 1953. "The age incidence of neural-arch defects in Alaskan natives, considered from the standpoint of etiology." *J. Bone Jt. Surg. (Amer.)* 35:937–950.

94. Troup, J. D. G. 1977. "The etiology of spondylolysis." *Orthop. Clin. N. Amer.* 8:57–64.

95. U.S. Social Security Disability Applicant Statistics. 1973. Unpublished data.

96. Valkenburg, H. A., and Haanen, H. C. M. 1982. "The epidemiology of low back pain." In *Workshop on Idiopathic Low Back Pain.* St. Louis: The C. V. Mosby Co. In press.

97. Ward, T., Knowelden, J., and Sharrand, W. J. W. 1968. "Low back pain." *J. Roy. Coll. Gen. Pract.* 15:128–136.

98. Waris, W. 1948. "Lumbar disc herniation, clinical studies and late results of 374 cases of sciatica." *Acta Chir. Scand Suppl.* 140.

99. White, A. A., and Panjabi, M. M. 1978. *The Clinical Biomechanics of the Spine.* Philadelphia: Lippincott.

100. Wiltse, L. L. 1957. "Etiology of spondylolisthesis." *Clin. Orthop.* 10:48–60.

101. ———. 1962. "The etiology of spondylolisthesis." *J. Bone Jt. Surg. (Amer.)* 44:539–560.

102. ———, and Jackson, D. W. 1976. "Treatment of spondylolisthesis and spondylolysis in children." *Clin. Orthop.* 117:92–100.

103. ———, Newman, P. H., and Macnab, I. 1976. "Classification of spondylolysis and spondylolisthesis." *Clin. Orthop.* 117:23–29.

104. ———, Widell, E. H., Jr., and Jackson, D. W. 1975. "Fatigue fracture: The basic lesion in isthmic spondylolisthesis." *J. Bone Jt. Surg. (Amer.)* 57:17–22.

105. Wynne-Davies, R., and Scott, J. H. S. 1979. "Inheritance and spondylolisthesis, a radiographic family survey." *J. Bone Jt. Surg. (Brit.)* 61:301–305.

106. Yaskin, J. C., and Finkelstein, A. 1944. "Low-back and leg pains, some clinical considerations." *Clinics* 3:261–308.

107. Yoss, R. E., Corbin, K. B., MacCarty, C. S., and Love, J. G. 1957. "Significance of signs in localization of involved root in cervical disk protrusion." *Neurology* 7:673–683.

7 Disorders of the Extremities

Disorders of the extremities are a major cause of disability. They often affect people in their wage-earning years and thus have a large economic impact. Upper extremity disorders alone were estimated to cost over $10 billion in the United States in 1980 (50).

The most commonly occurring conditions affecting the extremities are arthritic disorders and acute injuries, both of which are covered elsewhere (see Chapters 4 and 8, respectively). The first four disorders included in this chapter—carpal tunnel syndrome, Dupuytren's contracture, de Quervain's disease, and Volkmann's ischemic contracture—usually affect the upper extremities, while flat foot, osteochondritis dissecans, and tears of the semilunar cartilage are primarily disorders of the lower extremities. Although these conditions are frequently seen in clinical practice, little reliable information is available on their frequency in the general population. Few epidemiologic studies have been undertaken, and it will readily be seen that many clinical observations need to be followed up by more systematic epidemiologic study.

CARPAL TUNNEL SYNDROME

The carpal tunnel syndrome is a disorder of the wrist in which the median nerve is compressed against the transverse carpal ligament as it passes from the forearm into the hand (see Figure 7-1). The compression occurs within the carpal tunnel, which is surrounded by carpal bones on three sides and the transverse carpal ligament on the fourth. The usual

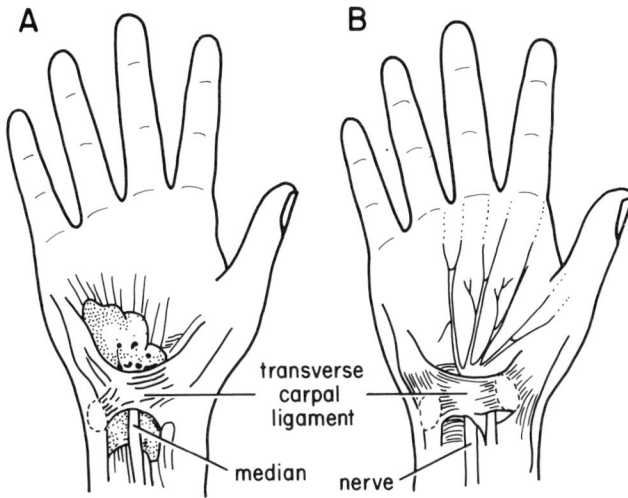

Figure 7-1   Carpal tunnel.

Source: Tobin (95). Reprinted with permission from *Amer. J. Obstet. and Gynec.,* Vol. 97, 1967, p. 494.

symptoms are pain, numbness, tingling or a prickling sensation in the palmar aspect of the thumb, index, and middle fingers and the radial side of the ring finger, this corresponding to the area supplied by the median nerve. In some patients, the pain radiates to the shoulder and neck as well. The symptoms tend to be worse at night. The condition is found bilaterally in about 55 percent of cases; the dominant hand tends to be the first and most severely affected (21,30,44,51,77,78,89,94,105). The ratio of cases with involvement of only the right wrist to cases with involvement of only the left has varied considerably from one study to another, but is probably at least 3 to 1.

Data are not available on the prevalence of the carpal tunnel syndrome in a defined population, although with the recent development of more sensitive diagnostic procedures and improved methods of treatment, it has been increasingly recognized as a common problem. The carpal tunnel syndrome occurs more often in women than in men, with reported ratios of females to males in different case series ranging from 2 to 1 to 6.6 to 1 (30,44,77,78,94,105). It is most frequently diagnosed in those 40 to 60 years of age (30,51,77,78,105); a slight excess frequency has occasionally been reported also at 25 to 30 years of age (30). The age distributions have apparently not been considered separately for males and females.

Familial aggregation of cases is slight. In families with several members affected, the condition is usually secondary to some other disorder, often appears in childhood, and has a male to female ratio of about 1 to 1 (22,34).

The carpal tunnel syndrome may be secondary to a variety of disorders, since any condition that increases the contents of the carpal canal may cause compression of the nerve against the transverse carpal ligament (13). For instance, the syndrome may result from a Colles' fracture of the wrist, either because the median nerve is caught between the fracture ends, or because of edema and swelling in the carpal tunnel (62). Rheumatoid arthritis is another frequently mentioned cause. Table 7-1 gives a list of disorders associated concomitantly with carpal tunnel syndrome in 915 cases seen at the Mayo Clinic from 1955 to 1961 (13). The conditions listed are fairly typical of those to which the carpal tunnel syndrome is attributed by practitioners. Whether all these disorders were actually responsible for the carpal tunnel syndrome is uncertain, since it is not known to what extent these percentages are greater than would be expected in a comparison group without the carpal tunnel syndrome. Other disorders associated by clinical impression with the carpal tunnel syndrome include acromegaly (74), infection of the arm and hand (9,101), amyloidosis (37), myeloma (38), hemophilia (52), and flexor dig-

Table 7-1 Conditions Associated with the Carpal Tunnel Syndrome Among 915 Cases Seen at the Mayo Clinic 1955-1961

Condition	Percentage of cases
Degenerative arthritis of cervical vertebrae or the involved wrist	18.4
Rheumatoid arthritis	10.5
Previous trauma	6.4
Diabetes	6.4
Localized tenosynovitis	5.4
Pregnancy	1.2
Gout	0.7
Periarthritis of shoulder	4.1
Thyroid disease	9.0
Other neurologic disorders	3.4
Hematologic diseases	1.7
Other miscellaneous disorders	2.2
No systemic disease	30.6

Source: Blodgett et al. (13).

itorum superficialis (2). Individuals on hemodialysis also have been reported to be at increased risk (45,48).

Thus, an unknown percentage of carpal tunnel syndrome cases is thought to be due to other disorders, but in many cases, no such predisposing conditions are found. Also, many people with these predisposing disorders do not develop the carpal tunnel syndrome, indicating that other factors are involved as well.

Repetitive hand motions, particularly those which involve flexion of the wrist and fingers, have long been thought to be associated with the development of the carpal tunnel syndrome. This belief arose in part because patients frequently complain of symptoms after strenuous or repetitive use of their hands (30,77,94,105) and in part because the higher frequency in women suggested that such activities as sewing, knitting, scrubbing, polishing, and writing were associated with an increased risk (30,51,77,94,105). In fact, one investigator (51) felt that the high frequency of the carpal tunnel syndrome during pregnancy occurred because of the greater amount of time devoted to knitting. Until recently, however, no really solid evidence existed to indicate that repetitive hand motions are involved in the etiology. Cannon et al. (18) have now reported from a small case-control study in a metal fabricating plant that cases are more likely than controls to have had jobs involving repetitive motion and jobs with exposure to vibration. Performance of tasks with the hands and wrists in awkward positions and exposure to vibration have also been suggested as etiologic factors on the basis of biomechanical analysis of jobs held by patients with the carpal tunnel syndrome (81).

The higher prevalence of the disorder in females has suggested a possible etiologic role for factors related to reproduction. The carpal tunnel syndrome has been observed to be very common during pregnancy (11,21,24,33,39,55,64,89,95,100), although there is disagreement about the time during pregnancy when the symptoms are most likely to begin. The symptoms usually disappear after the pregnancy unless permanent damage to the nerve has occurred (11,33,66,89); however, symptoms may remain as long as twenty months after pregnancy, and may reappear with subsequent pregnancies (74,95).

It is not known why the carpal tunnel syndrome should tend to appear with pregnancies. Clinical impressions suggest that fluid retention (24,39,77) and excessive weight gain early in pregnancy (100) may be the mechanisms, but other physicians (21,33) have not found these to be associated with the carpal tunnel syndrome in their patients. Poor posture during pregnancy has been hypothesized to put excessive strain on the cervical nerve, which in turn produces symptoms of the carpal tunnel syndrome (11,21), but again, this is based on clinical impression and has not been subjected to rigorous study. The hormone relaxin tends to result in fluid retention in the carpal tunnel; this could lead to symptoms (100), but there is disagreement (12) about the likelihood of this mechanism.

The high prevalence rate in women in the age group 40 to 60 years has suggested that menopause may be involved in the etiology. It has been hypothesized that induced menopause could precipitate the carpal tunnel syndrome (12), and that estrogen therapy could protect against it (55,80,84), but both of these suggestions were based on observations on small numbers of patients. Cannon (18), however, did find that gynecological surgery was reported more frequently in carpal tunnel syndrome cases than in controls. The possibility that oral contraceptives may be associated with the carpal tunnel syndrome because of fluid retention (83) also needs to be studied. Finally, there is disagreement as to whether a smaller carpal tunnel cross-sectional area is associated with an increased risk (2,23).

Thus, it is known that the carpal tunnel syndrome is most frequently diagnosed in females in the age range 40 to 60 years; also, it is likely that repetitive hand motions and perhaps vibration are involved in the etiology. Little else is known of the etiology of the carpal tunnel syndrome, unless some other disease such as a fracture or an arthritic disorder is the major cause. Various etiologic hypotheses have been suggested, many of which assume a role for fluid retention. Most of these hypotheses are derived from clinical impression, and it would seem that epidemiologic studies that tested these hypotheses would be the best way of adding to the rather limited body of current knowledge of the etiology of the carpal tunnel syndrome.

DUPUYTREN'S CONTRACTURE

Dupuytren's contracture is a disorder primarily affecting the hands. It consists of fibrosis and contracture of the palma fascia (fibrous tissue beneath the palm), resulting in flexion of the fingers at the metacarpophalangeal joints and the proximal interphalangeal joints (see Figure 7-2). Serious flexion deformity is usually limited to the ring and little fingers, but as the disease progresses the middle finger, index finger, and thumb can show moderate deformity. The disorder sometimes progresses to such an extent that the nails of the ring and little fingers dig into the palm. Occasionally, the plantar fascia of the foot is also involved.

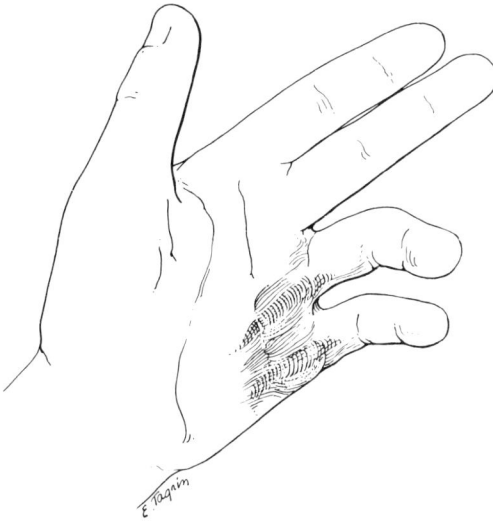

Figure 7-2 Dupuytren's contracture.

Source: MacAusland and Mayo (63).

Within the hand, the ring finger is most often affected by contracture, followed in frequency by the little finger, the middle finger, the thumb, and finally the index finger (14,16,68,106). The majority of cases are bilateral, but in unilateral cases the right hand is more often affected than the left in the ratio of approximately 2 to 1 (14,67,98,108). Among the bilateral cases, 10 percent or fewer develop contractures on both sides at the same time (69,108).

In a survey of a Norwegian population over 16 years of age, Dupuytren's contracture was present in 9 percent of men and 3 percent of women (67). Although hospital-based studies have indicated that over 50 percent of patients with Dupuytren's contracture are 40 to 59 years of age (14,97,98,108), the population-based Norwegian study indicated that prevalence rates increase steadily with age until finally dropping off in the 70 to 80 year age bracket (see Figure 7-3), and that the prevalence rate ranges from less than 2 percent among those under age 40 years to more than 30 percent in persons over 65 years. It is thus likely that surgical case series are overrepresented by people in their working years who are more likely to undergo surgical treatment.

Males are affected more frequently than females (14,26,67,87,98,108), although surgical case series inflate the true sex ratio, as shown by Mikkelsen's (68) finding that 6 percent of males but only 3 percent of females with Dupuytren's contracture in the general population had surgery for

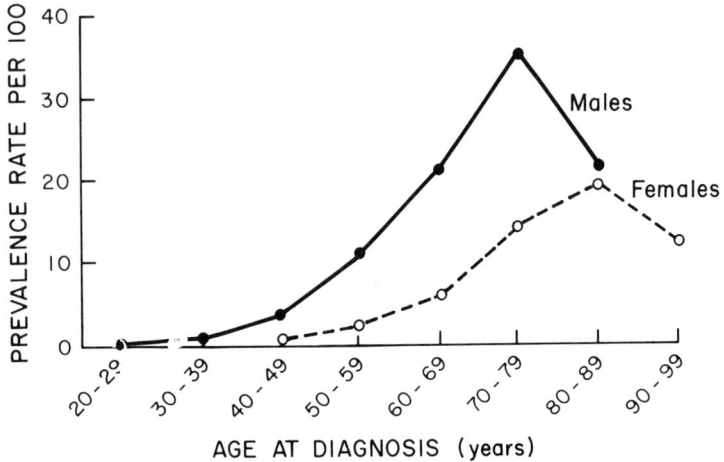

Figure 7-3   Prevalence per 100 of Dupuytren's disease in a Norwegian sample by sex and age at diagnosis. (−) men (−−−−) women.

Source: Mikkelsen (67).

their contracture. The best estimate of the male-to-female ratio is probably the 3 to 1 ratio found in Mikkelsen's general population survey.

Although it is generally believed that this disorder is more common in whites than blacks (106), it is not known whether this merely reflects the larger numbers of whites in the older high-risk age groups and the increased likelihood that the condition will be brought to medical attention and diagnosed among whites.

Factors other than age and sex that predispose to Dupuytren's contracture are not known. Possible risk factors that have perhaps received the most attention are manual labor, injuries, and heredity. Dupuytren himself believed that trauma was the main etiologic factor, but supporting evidence has not been forthcoming. Although Mikkelsen (70) reported that 24 percent of men with Dupuytren's contracture reported previous hand injuries compared to only 15 percent of normal men, people with hand deformity such as Dupuytren's contracture would be more likely to remember and report previous hand injuries than would those without such deformities. Table 7.2 shows the percentages of men and women with Dupuytren's contracture according to the extent of physical labor involved in their job. Although these data appear to suggest an etiologic role for heaviness of work, it is possible that workers with jobs requiring heavy physical activity are more likely to seek medical care for their problem than those with light or nonmanual jobs, so these results are difficult to interpret. Studies of occupational etiologic factors in Dupuytren's con-

Table 7.2

Type of work done	Percentage with Dupuytren's contracture	
	Men	Women
Heavy work	14.7	16.7
Moderately heavy work	11.4	3.1
Light manual work	9.5	2.8
Nonmanual work	5.3	0.9

Source: Mikkelson (70).

tracture are also made difficult by the tendency of many workers to change jobs once the condition develops (10).

Familial aggregation of cases has been suggested by a few authors (49,58) but not by all (97). Although this has been attributed to heredity, environmental factors could also explain the aggregation.

Another finding that may provide leads to etiology is an association between Dupuytren's contracture and epilepsy. An excess of Dupuytren's contracture has been found among epileptics (61,87), and a higher-than-expected prevalence of epilepsy has been reported among patients with Dupuytren's contracture (26,49). Mechanisms that have been suggested to explain these findings include a hereditary predisposition to both disorders, disturbances of the vasomotor system in epileptics, and side effects of treatments used for epilepsy. As yet, however, no strong evidence exists to support any of these possibilities.

Finally, an association between Dupuytren's contracture and heavy drinking of alcoholic beverages has been reported (46,82). Since it is likely that alcoholics differ from the general population in ways other than just their alcohol use, these data are not conclusive.

In summary, then, it has been established that Dupuytren's contracture is more common in males than in females, and that its prevalence increases with age. Beyond this, very little is known about its causation, although the possible role of manual labor and the association with epilepsy require further study.

DE QUERVAIN'S DISEASE

De Quervain's disease (stenosing tendovaginitis at the radial styloid) is a painful condition of the wrist in which there is thickening and narrowing of the tendon sheath where the extensor brevis and abductor pollicis longus tendons cross the styloid process at the lower end of the radius. The pain is usually localized to the styloid process (at the base of the thumb), although in some cases it may radiate into the hand or up the forearm. The pain is increased by abduction and extension of the thumb or by ulnar deviation of the hand. Weakness of the thumb and weakness of grip are also present. No data are available on prevalence rates for this disease.

Women are affected more frequently than men, such that about 85 to 90 percent of cases are female (25,73,107). The angle of the joint between the metacarpal and the radius is sharper in women than in men and is therefore more liable to trauma from friction (25). While the age at time of diagnosis may range from the middle teens to the middle seventies, almost half of diagnosed cases are between 40 and 60 years old (28).

In one case series (28) 53 percent of cases were found to be affected in the right wrist, 37 percent in the left wrist, and 10 percent were bilateral. It was also noted that among unilateral cases, 53 percent were affected in the dominant hand and 47 percent in the nondominant hand.

Anatomic anomalies in the extensor brevis and abductor pollicis longus pollicis tendons are frequently noted in patients with de Quervain's disease. Duthie and Ferguson (25), for instance, cite a series in which in 79 percent of cases, the abductor pollicis longus tendon was represented by two tendons, in 94 percent the extensor pollicis brevis tendon was very small, and in 33 percent the abductor pollicis longus occupied a separate compartment. These percentages are sufficiently high that one can conclude with some assurance that these anomalies of tendons do predispose to de Quervain's disease.

It is almost universally believed that de Quervain's disease results either from repeated mechanical trauma among people who use their thumb a great deal or from a single direct blow. Such manual activities as knitting, typing, operating a switchboard, playing the piano, golfing, and flycasting, in which the thumb in pinched while the wrist is moved, are thought to irritate the tendons and tendon sheaths (107). In an industrial plant, the following causes were most commonly reported: attempting a new kind of repetitive work, resuming repetitive work after a vacation or illness, doing repetitive work without any other special circumstance, direct blunt trauma to the wrist, and local "strain" (102). However, no epidemiologic data based on adequate sample size and appropriate comparison groups exist to support these impressions or case series reports. Thus, investigations are needed that focus on occupations at high risk and on the specific repetitive hand motions within these occupations that are associated with the elevated risk. Data should also be collected on cases in which medical care has not been sought since there are undoubtedly differences in the characteristics of people who seek medical attention for de Quervain's disease and those who do not.

VOLKMANN'S ISCHEMIC CONTRACTURE

This contracture is a shortening of certain muscles of the forearm such that there is a flexion deformity of the wrist and fingers and hyperextension of the metacarpal joints of all fingers (see Figure 7-4). The muscle contraction is caused by impedance of blood flow to these muscles, often in association with injury or obstruction to the brachial artery. Typically there is pain in the forearm, paleness in the fingers, prickling and tingling in the hand and arm, and paralysis of hand muscles. The degree to which the damage can be reversed depends in large part on the extent of the pathological lesion and the speed with which the cause of the contracture is corrected. The cause of the disorder may be any major fracture in the elbow, forearm, or upper arm, a contusion, or an overly tight bandage or plaster cast. Among patients treated for Volkmann's ischemic contracture

Figure 7-4   Volkmann's ischemic contracture.

Source: MacAusland and Mayo (63).

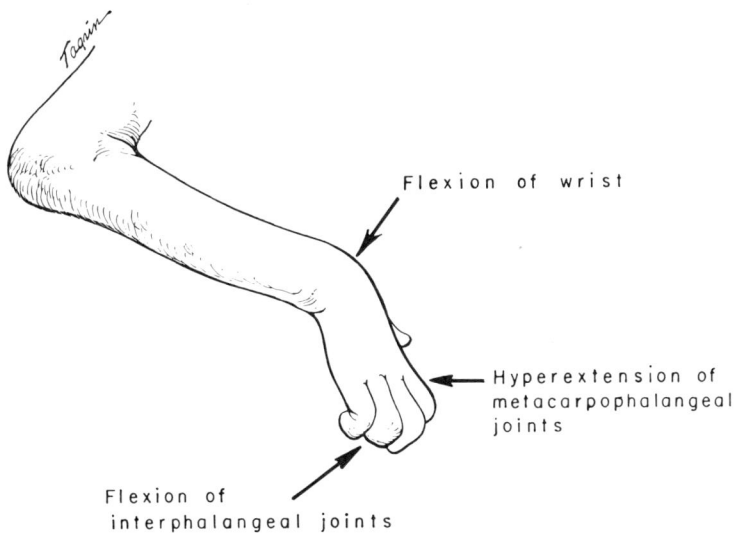

Flexion of wrist

Hyperextension of metacarpophalangeal joints

Flexion of interphalangeal joints

of the upper extremity at the Mayo Clinic during the years 1955 to 1965, about 35 percent were complications of supracondylar fractures around the elbow, and another 22 percent were complications of fractures of both bones of the forearm (27). An analogous contracture occurs in the lower limb, especially following fractures of the femoral shaft (72). The proportion of cases of iatrogenic origin has not been reported.

The frequency of Volkmann's contracture in a defined population is not known. According to a long-term study at the Mayo Clinic in Rochester, Minnesota, the proportion of admissions for patients with Volkmann's contracture has been declining since before 1935 (27). However, this trend can only be regarded as suggestive, since the value of the proportion would be influenced by its denominator as well as its numerator. This finding contrasts with a 20-year study in a Toronto children's hospital, which reported no change in the frequency of the contracture (72). While the two studies are not directly comparable, since the former included only patients with contractures of the forearm and the latter included patients with contractures of both the arm and the leg, the different conclusions reached by the two groups of investigators do indicate that not much is known for certain about trends in the incidence of this frequently preventable disorder.

Although the majority of cases of Volkmann's contracture occur in children, it has been found to occur in adults as well. Mayo Clinic study showed an average age of 22 years and a male-to-female ratio of more than 2 to 1 (27), the male excess probably corresponding to the greater frequency of injuries among males at young ages. In the same study, equal proportions of contractures were found to occur on the right and left sides. These findings, however, have not been corroborated and remain tentative.

FLAT FEET

In a flat foot, the longitudinal arch of the foot is lowered (see Figure 7-5). Normally the arch is preserved by the shape of the bones that comprise it, the plantar ligaments, and the tibial group of muscles. Flat feet may arise as a result of a weakness in any of these supporting elements and may occur congenitally or be acquired (25). In most cases flat feet cause no symptoms, but those that are painful make walking and participation in physical activities difficult.

Reviewing the epidemiology of flat foot is difficult because of the

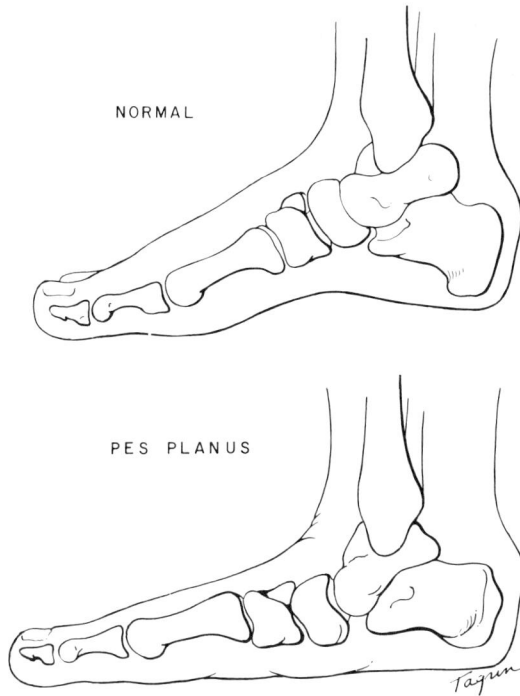

Figure 7-5   Normal foot and flat foot.

Source: MacAusland and Mayo (63).

absence of a standard accepted definition of what is a normal longitudinal arch and what is a flat foot, because of the different systems of classification of the various types of flat feet, and because the majority of flat feet cause no symptoms or disability while most studies focusing on etiology are based on cases seeking medical care. Diagnosing flat feet in infants and young children is particularly difficult. The feet of normal babies often appear flat because there is a fat pad in the instep. When infants begin to stand and walk, their feet may invert, but their feet may also turn out with apparent flattening, only to improve spontaneously as development proceeds. Preschool children may appear to have flat feet from an increase in ligamentous laxity, but around 6 years of age, the joints often tighten up and the flatness disappears (96). It is difficult at present to predict which feet will remain flat and which will not.

A survey of Canadian army recruits reported that 22.5 percent of men had feet that were considered flat or that had low arches. Other than this survey, very few studies of flat foot have been undertaken that could be considered epidemiologic, but the factors thought to be involved in the etiology of the different types of flat foot are reviewed here. In considering specific types of congenital flat feet, the classification given by Lovell et al. (60) will be used. Acquired flat feet will be discussed briefly later.

The first category of Lovell et al. (60) is congenital vertical talus (also called congenital convex pes planus, congenital rigid rocker-bottom foot, or congenital flat foot with talonavicular dislocation). In this condition, the sustentaculum tali is hypoplastic and does not provide adequate support for the head of the talus. This is a rigid type of flat foot, meaning that the foot is flat even when weight is not borne on it. Congenital vertical talus is rare, and its etiology is unknown. It may occur alone, but is frequently seen in combination with other congenital abnormalities such as congenital heart disease, foot deformities, vertebral stenosis, spinal cord lesions, spina bifida occulta, and arthrogryposis (19,32,43,53,59). It is usually bilateral (60), and is said to affect males more frequently than females (19,43,53,60). There is disagreement as to whether it aggregates in families (32,60). Various disorders have been suggested as possible causes, including disparity in growth between the muscles and bones of the lower leg (86), abnormal insertion of the tibialis anterior or overaction of the peroneal muscles (53), intrauterine compression from lack of space (53), laxity of muscles and ligaments (53), or arrest of the normal evolution of the tarsal region of the foot during the first four months of fetal life, particularly at the end of the second month and throughout the third month when the foot changes from a position in the same axis as the leg to a position that is supine relative to the leg (32). However, no strong evidence exists to support or refute any of these hypotheses.

Calcaneovalgus foot is a second type of flat foot seen in infants. This is a flexible form, meaning that the flatness is seen during weight bearing but not otherwise. In this type of flat foot, there is backward bending of the forefoot and hindfoot; if severe, the foot may be found lying against the anterior aspect of the tibia. It is bilateral in about 90 percent of cases (32). Calcaneovalgus flat feet are seen with considerably greater frequency than congenital vertical talus, but the prevalence rate is uncertain. Although familial aggregation definitely occurs, the pattern of inheritance is not clear (32).

A third type of congenital flat foot, termed flexible flat foot, is characterized by outward turning of the forefoot and heel, resulting in loss of the longitudinal arch during weight bearing; when weight is taken off the foot, the arch has a normal contour. This is often associated with generalized laxity of ligaments and is usually asymptomatic (60). No prevalence rates for this condition are available, and would depend greatly on the definition used. Debate about the etiology of this condition has been considerable, and has been reviewed by Lovell et al. (60). Harris and Beath (40,42), for instance, describe the "hypermobile flat foot with short tendo achillis," which they have found to be a clearly defined and particularly disabling type of flexible flat foot and which in Canadian army recruits had a prevalence rate of 6 percent. They believe that this condition results from weak support by the anterior portion of the calcaneus, that the relationship of the tarsal bones to one another affects its likelihood of occurrence, and that this condition is associated secondarily with a shortened Achilles tendon. Various investigators have felt that in particular the relationship of the os calcis to the talus is important in the etiology (60). Neurogenic and endocrine disorders have also been proposed as etiologic factors in flexible flat foot but have not been well studied (60).

The tarsal coalition, also sometimes called peroneal spastic flat foot, is a fourth type of congenital flat foot in which there is a union of two or more tarsal bones into a single structure. This condition almost always produces a rigid flat foot. The most common unions are a calcaneonavicular bar and a talocalcaneal bridge (99). Talonavicular, navicular cuneiform calcaneocuboid, and cubonavicular unions may also occur, as well as block coalitions. In all types the coalitions may be fibrous, cartilaginous, or osseous (20). The prevalence of this type of flat foot in Canadian male military recruits was found to be 2 percent (40,41). Usually people affected with the tarsal coalition do develop pain, which is aggravated by increased activity. Symptoms generally are noted during the second decade of life, apparently in association with rapid ossification (20). Often, the condition is unilateral (40). There is some familial aggregation of cases (60,99,104). Interestingly, Leonard (56) found in a survey of families of 31 patients with this disorder that 39 percent of relatives had some sort of tarsal coalition, but that none had had symptoms of the disorder. Proposed etiologic factors include the presence of an accessory bone that unites with the adjacent tarsal bone (41), abnormal growth changes in the foot (8), and errors in differentiation that may result in abnormalities ranging from complete bony fusion to an accessory bone that unites with adjacent tarsal bones (47).

Flat feet may be seen in adults either because they persisted from infancy or because they developed during adulthood. Good muscle bulk and tone are needed to support the bony arch of the foot during the adult years (5). Flat feet in adults are usually flexible and are in most instances asymptomatic. Proposed etiologic factors include (a) persistance of infantile flat foot because balancing muscles cannot be controlled and the foot collapses on weight bearing, (b) postural flat feet resulting from generalized poor muscle tone, (c) middle-aged flat feet resulting from a tendency for muscles to become flabby and for weight to be gained at this time of life, and (d) temporary flat feet, which may occur when weight bearing is resumed after muscles have lost their bulk or tone during prolonged illness without much weight bearing (e). There are also clinical impressions that occupations in which people must stand for long periods and vigorous exercise following periods when the feet are seldom used predispose to flat feet in adults (17,25). Contrary to popular opinion, there is no solid evidence that the type of footwear worn influences the likelihood of occurrence of flat feet. Finally, specific disorders such as fractures or diseases of bones of the feet or ruptures or avulsions of the plantar ligaments may result in acquired flat feet (25).

OSTEOCHONDRITIS DISSECANS

Osteochondritis dissecans is a localized disorder of joint surfaces in which a small segment of bone that has become avascular separates together with its covering articular cartilage from the rest of the bone to form a loose body in the joint space (see Figure 7-6). The only joint surfaces affected are convex ones to which tangential force can be applied. The distal femur (at the knee) is most frequently involved, followed by the lower end of the humerus. Less often, osteochondritis dissecans occurs in the heel, the superior aspect of the head of the femur, the head of the humerus, and the patella (5,31,36). Within the knee, between 70 and 85 percent of all lesions affect the medial femoral condyle, and only 15 to 30 percent occur in the lateral femoral condyle (4,36,57). About 10 percent of patients have osteochondritis dissecans at more than one site; often such lesions are symmetrical (36).

Although osteochondritis dissecans can affect an individual of any age, it usually occurs shortly after epiphyseal closure, that is, in late adolescence or young adulthood. The condition may be symptomless. In general, however, there are symptoms, which in the early stages usually consist of aching and swelling of the joint after exercise. If a loose body is formed, there will be recurrent sudden locking and unlocking of the joint; the locking occurs when the knee is in a variety of positions.

Cases of osteochondritis dissecans occur most frequently in individuals

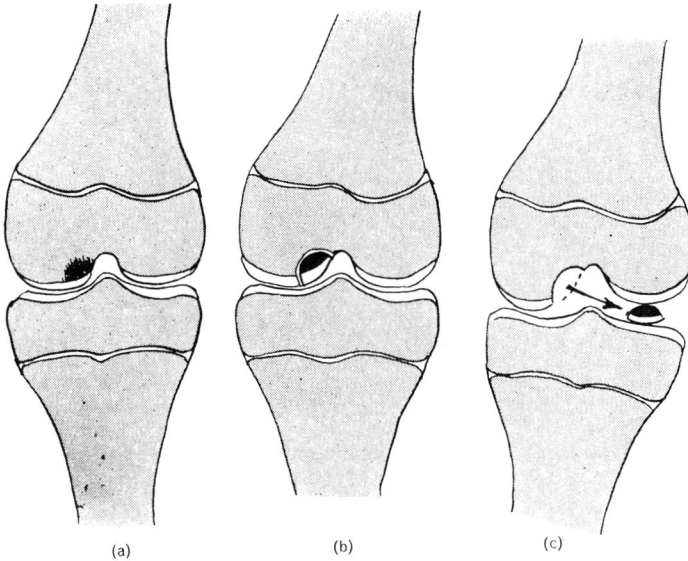

Figure 7-6 The formation of loose body in osteochondritis dissecans.
Source: Aston (7).

between 15 and 25 years of age. Boys are affected at least twice as often as girls, and the right side is involved slightly more often than the left (1,4,35,57,85,103).

In a study in Malmo, Sweden, from 1965 to 1974, age- and sex-specific incidence rates of osteochondritis dissecans of the femoral condyles among individuals seeking medical care were computed (see Figure 7-7) (57). In males, the annual incidence rate rose from about 2 per 100,000 at age 5 years to nearly 30 per 100,000 at age 15 years, then fell to 14 per 100,000 by age 25 years, and to about 10 per 100,000 at age 35 years. Females exhibited the same peak at 15 years of age, but the incidence rate at this age was only about 20 per 100,000. When the rates were considered for two time periods, 1965–69 and 1970–74, it was found that female rates remained at approximately 6 per 100,000 throughout both time periods, while the male rates increased from 9 to 15 per 100,000. One explanation for the increased incidence in males was the increased number of bone radiograms performed in the later period, but the female rate would have been expected to rise also. Another perhaps more reasonable explanation was that increased sports activity in the city had led to the increase in the number of injuries to the knee in males.

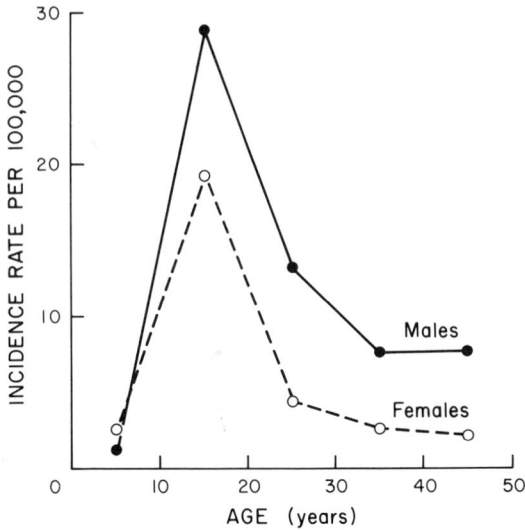

Figure 7-7   Sex- and age-specific incidence rates per 100,000 of osteochondritis dissecans in the femoral condyles in Malmo, Sweden.

Source: Linden (57).

   Many investigators believe that trauma is involved in the etiology, but there is debate about the mechanism by which trauma has its effect. It has generally been found that 40 to 55 percent of cases do report a recent history of significant knee injury (4,35). One study found that every one of eighteen young male patients with osteochondritis dissecans gave a history of organized athletic activity (15). However, no control group was used, and it is likely that this particular age and sex group has a high rate of participation in organized athletics. On the other hand, it has been pointed out that the areas of the body where this disorder most frequently occurs are relatively well protected from trauma. If trauma is involved, it therefore may be through multiple episodes of trauma having a thrombosing action on the blood vessels; this could cause ischemic necrosis, with acute trauma perhaps dislodging a bony fragment thus formed (1). Aichroth (3) produced osteochondral fractures in sixty rabbits, and found that nonunion of the fracture yielded a fragment that radiologically and histologically resembled osteochondritis dissecans. He concluded that the loose body in the joint is an ununited osteochondral fracture. Another experimental study in animals involved overloading the joints of twenty-two growing dogs and injecting the hormones somatotropin and thyrotropin into six of them (75). The dogs receiving mechanical trauma alone did not exhibit bone changes, but those receiving both mechanical trauma and hormones experienced changes in the articular cartilage and in the subchondral bone that were similar to those seen in spontaneous osteochondritis dissecans. These results suggest a combined hormonal and traumatic etiology that could together explain the observed age and sex distribution of cases.

Familial aggregation has also received attention. Families with several members affected have been reported (29,71,79,92,93). Some of these studies have included members of three or four generations, and an increased occurrence of osteochondritis dissecans of the knee and the elbow has been reported that is consistent with an autosomal dominant mode of inheritance (71,92,93). In contrast, Green (35) questioned 40 patients and found that none of them reported a family history of osteochondritis dissecans. Also, when eighty-six first-degree relatives of thirty-four patients were examined both clinically and radiologically, Petrie (76) found only one relative with the disease. Thus, although heredity may be important in some cases, in the majority of instances, heredity is probably not involved to any great extent.

Most investigators tend to consider repetitive trauma or perhaps single episodes of trauma as the most important etiologic factors, possibly in the presence of an underlying metabolic defect that may or may not be inherited.

TEARS OF THE SEMILUNAR CARTILAGE

Tears of the semilunar cartilage (meniscus) usually occur on the medial side of the knee, and most frequently result from a twisting strain on a flexed knee while a person is bearing weight. The semilunar cartilage is trapped between the femur and tibia, and when the leg is extended, the cartilage tears. Symptoms of torn cartilages include pain and swelling of the knee joint on the side of the tear, and sometimes locking of the joint, meaning that it cannot be fully extended. Tears on the medial side of the knee are much more common than on the lateral side because (a) the attachments of the lateral cartilage permit more mobility, (b) the lateral cartilage is less subject to shearing stress, and (c) severe internal twists on a flexed knee are less common than external twists (5,7).

No data are avilable on the frequency of torn semilunar cartilages in a defined population. However, during World War II, injuries of the semilunar cartilages were the most frequently diagnosed noncombat injury to military personnel, and meniscectomy (removal of semilunar cartilage) was the most common orthopedic operation among these personnel (91).

Young adults, particularly males, are affected most often (5,7). In a series of patients undergoing surgery for torn semilunar cartilages (90), 73 percent were males and 70 percent were under 40 years of age. Since the initial split of the cartilage requires (a) weight bearing, (b) a flexed knee, and (c) a twisting strain (5), sports in which there may be a sudden twist of the knee, such as football, are most frequently associated with these injuries. In certain occupations such as mining, the risk of tears of the semilunar cartilage is also high. Miners often have to work while stooping or squatting and have to twist while in this position. If they twist at the level of the knee, the cartilage may become entrapped and if the leg is suddenly extended, the cartilage may tear (7,25,88).

In 42 percent of patients seen in the case series mentioned previously (90), no traumatic event was reported to have preceded the knee pain, so that sudden single episodes of twisting are by no means the only cause. In fact, in people over 30 years of age, degenerative changes appear to be more important than any single injury (88). Occupations that require prolonged squatting or kneeling may bring about degenerative changes such that only a minor motion of the knee may lead to detachment of the cartilage. Also, small initial tears may become enlarged with continued stress on them (54).

Other suggested predisposing factors are laxity of the meniscal attachments to the capsule, poor fibrocartilage, muscle weakness, poor mechanics of the knee such as would result from previous ligamentous injuries, ligamentous laxity of the joint, obesity, and congenital anomalies of the menisci (54,88,91). Circumstantial evidence suggesting that weakness of muscles, ligaments, and other periarticular structures predisposes to injuries of semilunar cartilage dates back to the observation made during the Mesopotamian campaign of World War I that large numbers of injuries occurred in autumn, when physical activity was resumed after all hostilities and strenuous exercises had temporarily ceased during the summer months (65).

In summary, the etiologic role of sudden twisting strains on a flexed knee is well established. However, more investigation is needed of the factors contributing to torn semilunar cartilages when there is no one single precipitating episode and of factors that make one person's knee more susceptible than another when single episodes of trauma are involved.

REFERENCES

1. Aegerter, E., and Kirkpatrick, J. A., Jr. 1975. *Orthopaedic Diseases.* Philadelphia: Saunders.
2. Aghasi, M. K., Rzetelny, V., and Axer, A. 1980. "The flexor digitorum superficialis as a cause of bilateral carpal-tunnel syndrome and trigger wrist." *J. Bone Jt. Surg.* 62:134–135.
3. Aichroth, P. 1971. "Osteochondral fractures and their relationship to osteochondritis dissecans of the knee. An experimental study in animals." *J. Bone Jt. Surg. (Brit.)* 53:448–454.
4. ———. 1971. "Osteochondritis dissecans of the knee—A clinical survey." *J. Bone Jt. Surg. (Brit.)* 53:440–447.
5. Apley, A. G. 1977. *A System of Orthopaedics and Fractures.* London: Butterworths.
6. Armstrong, T. J., and Chaffin, D. B. 1979. "Carpal tunnel syndrome and selected personal attributes." *J. Occup. Med.* 21:481–486.
7. Aston, J. N. 1967. *A Short Textbook of Orthopaedics and Traumatology.* Philadelphia: Lippincott.
8. Badgley, C. E. 1927. "Coalition of the calcaneus and the navicular." *Arch. Surg.* 15:75–88.
9. Bailey, D., and Carter, J. F. B. 1955. "Median-nerve palsy associated with acute infections of the hand." *Lancet* 1:530–532.
10. Bell, R. C., and Furness, J. A. 1977. "A study of the effect of recurrent trauma on the development of Dupuytren's contracture." *Brit. J. Plast. Surg.* 30:149–150.
11. Benson, R. C., and Inman, V. T. 1956. "Brachialgia statica dysesthetica in pregnancy." *Wes. J. Surg.* 64:115–130.
12. Bjorkquist, S. E., Lang, A.H., Punnoner, R., and Rauramo, L. 1977. "Carpal tunnel syndrome in ovariectomized women." *Acta Obstet. Gynecol. Scand.* 56:127–130.
13. Blodgett, R. C., Lipschomb, P. R., and Hill, R. W. 1962. "Incidence of hematologic disease in patients with carpal tunnel syndrome." *J. Amer. Med. Asso.* 182:814–815.
14. Boyes, J. H. 1954. "Dupuytren's contracture: Notes on the age at onset and the relationship to handedness." *Amer. J. Surg.* 88:147–154.
15. Brown, R., Blazina, M. E., Kerlan, R. K., Carter, V. S., Jobe, F. W., and Carlson, G. J. 1974. "Osteochondritis of the capitellum." *J. Sports Med.* 2:27–46.
16. Bruner, J. M. 1970. "The dynamics of Dupuytren's disease." *Hand* 2:172–177.
17. Caillet, R. 1968. *Foot and Ankle Pain.* Philadelphia: Saunders.
18. Cannon, L. J., Bernacki, E. J., and Walter, S. D. 1981. "Personal and occupational factors associated with the carpal tunnel syndrome." *J. Occup. Med.* 23:255–258.
19. Coleman, S. S., Stelling, F. H. III, and Jarrett, J. 1970. "Pathomechanics and treatment of congenital vertical talus." *Clin. Orthop.* 70:62–72.
20. Conway, J. J., and Cowell, H. R. 1969. "Tarsal coalition: Clinical significance and roentgenographic demonstration." *Radiology* 92:799–811.
21. Crisp, W. E., and DeFrancesco, S. 1964. "The hand syndrome of pregnancy." *Obstet. and Gynec.* 23:433–437.
22. Danta, G. 1975. "Familial carpal tunnel syndrome with onset in childhood." *J. Neurol., Neurosurg., Psych.* 38:350–355.
23. Dekel, S., and Coates, R. 1979. "Primary carpal stenosis as a cause of 'idiopathic' carpal-tunnel syndrome." *Lancet* 2:1024.
24. Downie, A. W. 1964. "Carpal tunnel syndrome during pregnancy." *J. Amer. Med. Asso.* 190:689.

25. Duthie, R. B., and Ferguson, A. B., Jr. 1973. *Mercer's Orthopaedic Surgery.* London: Arnold.
26. Early, P. F. 1962. "Population studies in Dupuytren's contracture." *J. Bone Jt. Surg. (Brit.)* 44:602–613.
27. Eichler, G. R., and Lipscomb, P. R. 1967. "The changing treatment of Volkmann's ischemic contractures from 1955 to 1965 at the Mayo Clinic." *Clin. Orthop.* 50:215–223.
28. Faithfull, D. K., and Lamb, D. W. 1971, "De Quervain's disease—A clinical review." *Hand* 3:23–30.
29. Gardiner, T. B. 1955. "Osteochondritis dissecans in three members of one family." *J. Bone Jt. Surg. (Brit.)* 37:137–141.
30. Garland, H., Bradshaw, T. P. P., and Clark, J. M. P. 1957. "Compression of median nerve in carpal tunnel and its relation to acroparesthesia." *Brit. Med. J.* 1:730–734.
31. Gartland, J. J. 1974. *Fundamentals of Orthopaedics.* Philadelphia: Saunders.
32. Giannestras, N. J. 1970. "Recognition and treatment of flat feet in infancy." *Clin. Orthop.* 70:10–29.
33. Gould, J. S., and Wissinger, H. A. 1978. "Carpal tunnel syndrome in pregnancy." *South Med. J.* 71:144–145.
34. Gray, R. G., Poppo, M. J., and Gottlieb, N. L. 1979. "Primary familial bilateral carpal tunnel syndrome." *Ann. Int. Med.* 91:37–40.
35. Green, J. P. 1966. "Osteochondritis dissecans of the knee." *J. Bone Jt. Surg. (Brit.)* 48:82–91.
36. Griffin, P. P. 1978, "The lower limb." In *Pediatric Orthopaedics.* W. W. Lovell and R. B. Winter, eds. Philadelphia: Lippincott, pp. 881–909.
37. Grokoest, A. W., and Demactini, F. E. 1954. "Systemic disease and the carpal tunnel syndrome." *J. Amer. Med. Asso.* 155:635–637.
38. Grossman, L. A., Kaplan, H. J., Ownby, F. D., and Grossman, M. 1961. "Carpal tunnel syndrome—Initial manifestation of systemic disease." *J. Amer. Med. Asso.* 176:259–261.
39. Guly, P. J. 1959. "Carpal tunnel syndrome," (letter). *Brit. Med. J.* 1:1184.
40. Harris, R. I., and Beath, T. 1947. *Army Foot Survey.* National Research Council of Canada. Ottawa.
41. ———, and Beath, T. 1948. "Etiology of peroneal spastic flat foot." *J. Bone Jt. Surg. (Brit.)* 30:624–634.
42. ———, and Beath, T. 1948. "Hypermobile flat foot with short tendo achillis." *J. Bone Jt. Surg. (Amer.)* 30:116–140.
43. Harrold, A. J. 1967. "Congenital vertical talus in infancy." *J. Bone Jt. Surg. (Brit.)* 49:634–643.
44. Heathfield, K. W. G. 1957. "Acroparaesthesia and the carpal-tunnel syndrome." *Lancet* 2:663–666.
45. Holtmann, B., and Anderson, C. B. 1977. "Carpal tunnel syndrome following vascular shunts for hemodialysis." *Arch. Surg.* 112:65–66.
46. Hueston, J. T. 1960. "The incidence of Dupuytren's contracture." *Med. J. Aust.* 2:999–1002.
47. Jack, E. A. 1954. "Bone anomalies of the tarsus in relation to 'peroneal spastic flat foot'." *J. Bone Jt. Surg. (Brit.)* 36:530–542.
48. Jain, V. J. K., Cestero, R. V. M., and Baum, J. 1979. "Carpal tunnel syndrome in patients undergoing maintenance hemodialysis." *J. Amer. Med. Ass.* 242:2868–2869.
49. James, J. I. P. 1969. "The relationship of Dupuytren's contracture and epilepsy." *Hand* 1:47–49.

50. Kelsey, J. L., Pastides, H., Kreiger, N., Harris, C., and Chernow, R. A. 1980. *Upper Extremity Disorders, A Survey of Their Frequency and Cost in the United States.* St. Louis: C. V. Mosby Co.
51. Kendall, D. 1960. "Aetiology, diagnosis, and treatment of paraesthesia in the hands." *Brit. Med. J.* 2:1633–1640.
52. Khunadorn, N., Schlagenhauss, R. E., Tourbaf, K., and Papademetrion, T. 1977. "Carpal tunnel syndrome in hemophilia." *N.Y. State J. Med.* 77:1314–1315.
53. Lamy, L., and Weissman, L. 1939. "Congenital convex pes valgus." *J. Bone Jt. Surg.* 21:79–91.
54. Larson, R. L. 1975. "Dislocations and ligamentous injuries of the knee." In *Fractures.* C. A. Rockwood, Jr. and D. P. Green, eds. Philadelphia: Lippincott, pp. 1182–1284.
55. Layton, R. B. 1958. "Acroparesthesia in in pregnancy and the carpal-tunnel syndrome." *J. Obstet. and Gynec. Brit. Emp.* 65:823–825.
56. Leonard, M. A. 1974. "The inheritance of tarsal coalition and its relationship to spastic flat foot." *J. Bone Jt. Surg. (Brit.)* 56:520–526.
57. Linden, B. 1976. "The incidence of osteochondritis dissecans in the condyles of the femur." *Acta Orthop. Scand.* 47:664–667.
58. Ling, R. S. M. 1963. "The genetic factor in Dupuytren's disease." *J. Bone Jt. Surg. (Brit.)* 45:709–718.
59. Lloyd-Roberts, G. G., and Spence, A. J. 1958. "Congenital vertical talus." *J. Bone Jt. Surg. (Brit.)* 40:33–41.
60. Lovell, W. W., Price, C. T., and Meehan, P. L. 1978. "The foot." In *Pediatric Orthopaedics.* W. W. Lovell and R. B. Winter, eds. Philadelphia: Lippincott, pp. 911–997.
61. Lund, M. 1941. "Dupuytren's contracture and epilepsy." *Acta Psych. Neurol.* 16:465–492.
62. Lynch, A. C., and Lipscomb, P. R. 1963. "The carpal tunnel syndrome and Colles fractures." *J. Amer. Med. Ass.* 185:363–366.
63. MacAusland, W. R., Jr., and Mayo, R. A. 1965. *Orthopedics.* Boston: Little Brown, and Company.
64. Massey, E. W. 1978. "Carpal tunnel syndrome in pregnancy." *Obstet. Gynecol. Surv.* 33:145–148.
65. McNeill Love, R. J. 1923. "Prognosis after removal of semilunar cartilages." *Brit. Med. J.* 2:324–326.
66. Melvin, J. L., Burnett, C. N., and Johnson, E. W. 1969. "Median nerve conduction in pregnancy." *Arch of Phys. Med. Rehab.* 50:75–80.
67. Mikkelsen, O. A. 1972. "The prevalence of Dupuytren's disease in Norway." *Acta Chir. Scand.* 138:695–700.
68. ———. 1976. "Dupuytren's disease—A study of the pattern of distribution and stage of contracture in the hand." *Hand* 8:265–271.
69. ———. 1977. "Dupuytren's disease—Inital symptoms, age of onset and spontaneous course." *Hand* 9:11–15.
70. ———. 1978. "Dupuytren's disease—The influence of occupation and previous hand injuries." *Hand* 10:1–8.
71. Mubarak, S. J., and Carroll, N. C. 1979. "Familial osteochondritis dissecans of the knee." *Clin. Orthop.* 140:131–136.
72. ———, and Carroll, N. C. 1979, "Volkmann's contracture in children: Aetiology and prevention." *J. Bone Jt. Surg. (Brit.)* 61:285–293.
73. Muckart, R. D. 1964. "Stenosing tendovaginitis of abductor pollicis longus and extensor pollicis brevis at the radial styloid (de Quervain's disease)." *Clin. Orthop.* 33:201–208.

74. O'Duffy, J. D., Randall, R. V., and MacCarty, C. S. 1973. "Median neuropathy (carpal-tunnel syndrome) in acromegaly. A sign of endocrine overactivity." *Ann. Int. Med.* 78:379–383.
75. Paatsama, S., Rokkanen, P., and Jussila, J. 1975. "Etiological factors in osteochondritis dissecans. An experimental study in the etiological factors in osteochondritis dissecans in the canine humeral head using overloading with and without somatotropin and thyrotropin hormone treatment and mechanical trauma." *Acta Orthop. Scand.* 46:906–918.
76. Petrie, P. W. R. 1977. "Aetiology of osteochondritis dissecans. Failure to establish a familial background." *J. Bone Jt. Surg. (Brit.)* 59:366–367.
77. Phalen, G. S. 1966. "The carpal-tunnel syndrome. 17 years experience with 654 hands." *J. Bone Jt. Surg. Amer.* 48:211–228.
78. ———. 1972. "The carpal-tunnel syndrome." *Clin. Orthop.* 83:29–40.
79. Pick, M. P. 1955. "Familial osteochondritis dissecans." *J. Bone Jt. Surg. (Brit.)* 37:142–145.
80. Reid, S. F. 1956. "Tenovaginitis stenosis at the carpal tunnel." *Aust. New Zeal. J. Surg.* 25:204–213.
81. Rothfleisch, S., and Sherman, D. 1978. "Carpal tunnel syndrome. Biomechanical aspects of occupational occurrence and implications regarding surgical management." *Orthop. Rev.* 7:107–109.
82. Sabiston, D. W. 1973. "Cataracts, Dupuytren's contracture, and alcohol addiction." *Amer. J. Ophthal.* 76:1005–1007.
83. Sabour, M. S., and Fadel, H. E. 1970. "The carpal tunnel syndrome—A new complication ascribed to the pill." *Amer. J. Obstet. Gynecol.* 107:1265–1267.
84. Schiller, F., and Kolb, F. O. 1954. "Carpal tunnel syndrome in acromegaly." *Neurology* 4:271–282.
85. Scott, D. J., and Stevenson, C. A. 1971. "Osteochondritis dissecans of the knee in adults." *Clin. Orthop.* 76:82–86.
86. Silk, F. F., and Wainwright, D. 1967. "The recognition and treatment of congenital flatfoot in infancy." *J. Bone Jt. Surg. (Brit.)* 49:628–633.
87. Skoog, T. 1948. "Dupuytren's contraction with special reference to aetiology and improved surgical treatment, its occurrence in epileptics, note on knuckle-pads." *Acta Chir. Scand. Suppl.* 139:1–190.
88. Smillie, I. S. 1980. *Injuries of the Knee Joint.* Edinburgh: Churchill Livingstone.
89. Soferman, N., Weissman, S. L., and Haimov, M. 1964. "Acroparesthesias in pregnancy." *Amer. J. Obstet. and Gynec.* 89:528–531.
90. Stenstrom, A., Hagstedt, B., Hansson, L. I., and Ljung, P. 1978. "Meniscectomy A comparison of two series treated as outpatients and inpatients." *Acta Orthop. Scand.* 49:403–406.
91. Stewart, M. 1971. "Traumatic affections of joints." In *Campell's Operative Orthopaedics.* A. H. Crenshaw, ed. St. Louis: The C. V. Mosby Co., pp. 901–962.
92. Stougaard, J. 1961. "The hereditary factor in osteochondritis dissecans." *J. Bone Jt. Surg. (Brit.)* 43:256–258.
93. ———. 1964. "Familial occurrence of osteochondritis dissecans." *J. Bone Jt. Surg. (Brit.)* 46:542–543.
94. Tanzer, R. C. 1959. "The carpal-tunnel syndrome." *J. Bone Jt. Surg.* 41:626–634.
95. Tobin, S. M. 1967. "Carpal tunnel syndrome in pregnancy." *Amer. J. Obstet. and Gynec.* 97:493–498.
96. Walker, G. 1972. "Orthopaedic problems of childhood." *Practitioner* 208:227–238.

97. Wallace, A. F. 1965. "Dupuytren's contracture in women." *Brit. J. Plast. Surg.* 18:385–386.
98. Wang, M. K. H., Macomber, W. B., Stein, A., Rajpal, R., and Heffernan, A. 1960. "Dupuytren's contracture. An analytic and etiologic study." *Plast. Reconstr. Surg.* 25:323–336.
99. Webster, F. S., and Roberts, W. M. 1951. "Tarsal anomalies and peroneal spastic flatfoot." *J. Amer. Med. Ass.* 146:1099–1104.
100. Wilkinson, M. 1960. "The carpal-tunnel syndrome in pregnancy." *Lancet* 1:453–454.
101. Williams, L. F., and Geer, T. 1963. "Acute carpal tunnel syndrome secondary to pyogenic infection of the forearm." *J. Amer. Med. Ass.* 185:409–410.
102. Wilson, R. N., and Wilson, S. 1957. "Tenosynovitis in industry." *Practitioner* 178:612–625.
103. Woodward, A. H., and Bianco, A. J. 1975. "Osteochondritis dissecans of the elbow." *Clin. Orthop.* 110:35–41.
104. Wray, J. B., and Herndon, C. N. 1963. "Hereditary transmission of congenital coalition of the calcaneus to the navicular." *J. Bone Jt. Surg. (Amer.)* 45:365–372.
105. Yamaguski, D. M., Lipscomb, P. R., and Sonle, E. H. 1965. "Carpal tunnel syndrome." *Minn. Med.* 48:22–33.
106. Yost, J., Winters, T., and Fett, H. C. 1955. "Dupuytren's contracture—A statistical study." *Amer. J. Surg.* 90:568–574.
107. Younghusband, O. Z., and Black, J. D. 1963. "De Quervain's disease: Stenosing tenovaginitis of the radial styloid process." *Can. Med. Assoc. J.* 89:508–512.
108. Zachariae, L. 1971. "Dupuytren's contracture: The aetiological role of trauma." *Scand. J. Plast. Reconstr. Surg.* 5:116–119.

8 Acute Musculoskeletal Injuries

Among the common acute injuries to the musculoskeletal system are fractures, dislocations, strains, and sprains. Fracture refers to the breaking of a bone, dislocation to the displacement of a bone, sprain to the wrenching of a joint with partial rupture or other injury of its attachments, and strain to the overstretching or overexertion of some part of the musculature. The frequency of occurrence of these four types of injuries will first be presented as well as the usual mechanisms of injury for the most commonly occurring sprains and dislocations. Since fractures are generally the most serious of these injuries, they will then be discussed in more detail.

There are various other types of acute musculoskeletal injuries, many of which are discussed elsewhere in this book. In particular, some of the conditions discussed in Chapters 6 and 7 on disorders of the back and neck and extremities may have a sudden onset following episodes of physical trauma. Injuries to the spinal cord will not be considered except to mention that although they are uncommon, they are associated with much physical and emotional trauma and involve enormous costs. The majority of incident cases occur in males in the age range 16 to 35 years, and motor vehicle accidents are the leading cause (18,19).

FRACTURES, DISLOCATIONS, SPRAINS, AND STRAINS: GENERAL ASPECTS

Data from the Health Interview Survey of the National Center for Health Statistics (23) indicate that each year an average of 1 of every 10 persons in the United States suffers a fracture, dislocation, sprain, or strain of sufficient severity to warrant medical care or activity restriction. Table 8-1 shows age-specific annual incidence rates for the four conditions combined, at this level of severity. These fractures and dislocations are on the average associated with about three weeks of restricted activity and almost one week in bed per episode (Table 8-2). However, about two-thirds of the acute musculoskeletal injuries for which medical care is sought or activity restricted are sprains and strains, which are on the average associated with only about one week of restricted activity and one to two days in bed per episode.

Estimates of the number of injuries in a year in the United States for the most common sites of strains and sprains are given in Table 8-3. The back is most frequently affected, followed by the ankle and foot, then the knee and leg. Strains and sprains of the back occur most often in individuals of working age. Estimates indicate that each year nearly 1 out of 30 individuals in the age range 17 to 64 years has a strain or sprain of the back sufficiently severe to warrant medical care or restriction of activity (24,33). Further information on injuries to the back is found in Chapter 6. Strains and sprains of the ankle and foot are almost as frequent, and most often occur in the 6 to 16 year age group, primarily because of the large amount of physical activity of individuals in this age span (34). Sprains of the ankle generally result from internal rotational injuries, and the lateral ligament is most frequently damaged (4).

Injuries to the ligaments of the knee most commonly occur in young adults and usually involve the medial ligament; the injury generally

Table 8-1 Incidence per 100 of Fractures and Dislocations and Sprains and Strains to the Musculoskeletal System, United States, July 1975–June 1976, by Age

Age (in years)	Incidence per 100		
	Fractures and dislocations	Sprains and strains	Total
<6	1.3	1.0	2.3
6–16	4.3	7.2	11.5
17–44	2.8	9.9	12.7
≥45	2.9	4.1	7.0
All ages	3.0	6.8	9.8

Source: National Center for Health Statistics (24) for numerators, U.S. Bureau of the Census (33) for denominators.

Table 8-2 Average Number of Days of Restricted Activity and Bed Disability per Traumatic Episode for Fractures and Dislocations, Sprains and Strains to the Musculoskeletal System, United States, July 1975–June 1976, by Age

Age (in years)	Fractures and dislocations	Sprains and strains	Total
Average number of restricted days			
<6	6.9	1.2	4.5
6–16	18.8	2.9	8.9
17–44	19.5	6.2	9.2
≥45	27.9	10.5	17.7
All ages	21.3	6.3	10.9
Average number of bed days			
<6	2.4	1.0	1.8
6–16	2.8	0.6	1.4
17–44	6.5	1.7	2.8
≥45	9.2	2.2	5.1
All ages	6.1	1.6	3.0

Source: National Center for Health Statistics (24).

Table 8-3 Estimated Average Annual Number of New Cases of Strains and Sprains Associated with a Visit to a Physician or with Restriction of Activity, Five Most Common Sites, United States, 1975–1976

Site	Number
Back	4,938,000
Ankle and foot	4,686,000
Knee and leg	1,893,000
Wrist and hand	1,564,000
Shoulder and upper arm	843,000

Source: National Center for Health Statistics (24).

occurs when the knee is in extension and is suddenly subjected to unexpected force. Such injuries are particularly common in football, but also occur frequently in skiing, soccer, basketball, gymnastics and wrestling, as well as in industrial, home, and motor vehicle accidents (21).

Dislocations are less common than strains, sprains, or fractures. In fact, site-specific data from the Health Interview Survey are not considered reliable by the National Center for Health Statistics because of the relatively small number of people reporting these injuries. Keeping in mind the wide margins of errors associated with the estimates, the most frequently affected sites appear to be the shoulder, elbow, wrist, finger, hip, and knee (24).

Dislocated shoulders may affect individuals of any age, but are most often recurrent and therefore disabling in persons under age 20 years (Table 8-4) (27). Anterior dislocations are much more common than posterior dislocations, and usually result from trauma, particularly from falls on the hand with the arm abducted or from direct blows to the shoulder. Forceful motion with the arm in extension, in elevation, or in external

Table 8-4   Age of Patient at the Time of Primary Shoulder
Dislocation in Relation to the Incidence of Recurrence

Age of patient (years)	Number of primary dislocations	Number of recurrences	Incidence of recurrence
1–10	4	4	100%
11–20	49	46	94%
21–30	64	51	79%
31–40	16	8	50%
41–50	33	8	24%
51–60	63	9	14%
61–70	50	8	16%
71–80	32	2	6%
81–90	10	0	0%
	321	136	42%
Total shoulders*	324		
Under 20 years			94% recurred
20–40			74
Over 40			14

*(3 bilateral cases)

Source: Rowe (27).

rotation may also bring about dislocations (4,28). For recurrent dislocations, less force may be required with each successive episode (4,8,30).
Although rare, voluntary dislocation also may occur in adolescents and
young adults when one group of muscles is contracted and the antagonist
group suppressed (29).

Elbow dislocations occur in both children and adults. Posterior dislocations usually result from falls on an outstretched hand with the arm in
extension while anterior dislocations commonly occur from a blow to a
flexed elbow (9). Among finger dislocations, posterior dislocations of both
the proximal and distal interphalangeal joint are most common; these
dislocations result from hyperextension of the joint, such as when an outstretched finger is struck with a ball (3,13).

FRACTURES

Fractures of bone occur when stress produced by forces applied to bone
exceeds the breaking stress of the bone. As indicated in the previous section, fractures usually restrict activity for about three weeks and, at least
in the young, are often not regarded as particularly disabling in the long
run, unless associated with other serious injuries such as spinal cord
trauma. However, the extent of disability is much greater among the
elderly. For example, hip fractures, one of the most common serious injuries in the elderly, are associated with a great deal of morbidity and mortality (10). Even among a group of women of age 55 and over who were
considered to be at "good risk" for undergoing surgical pinning of their
hips, a study indicated that fewer than one-quarter had gained full recovery at six months after the fracture (7). Over half needed assistance to
walk and carry on their usual activities, while about one-quarter could
neither walk nor carry on their usual activities even with assistance.

The forces to which bone is exposed and the breaking stress of bone
differ between males and females and by age group. Considering fractures of all sites combined, incidence rates generally increase with age,
although the increase is considerably less for males than for females. At
young ages, fractures occur more commonly in males than females. The
male-to-female ratio changes sharply with increasing age, and by 85
years of age females are twice as likely to incur a fracture as males (17).
In males, the age group with the highest fracture rate is the 15 to 24 year
age group, while for females, fracture rates are highest in the 65 and older
age groups (16). At young ages, excessive force applied to bone from

severe trauma is important etiologically, whereas at older ages, brittleness of bone associated with osteoporosis is a major factor. With increasing age, a greater proportion of fractures of long bones such as the humerus, ulna, and femur involve the spongy end of these bones (the metaphysis) rather than the bone shaft (diaphysis), since the osteoporotic process generally affects the spongy trabecular bone to a greater extent than the compact cortical bone of the shaft (2,6,11).

Reliable data on the frequency with which various bones are fractured apparently are not available. Most reports are based on cases seen at hospitals, but fractures of many sites are often treated in physicians' offices rather than in hospitals. Perhaps the only usable data are derived from the U.S. Health Interview Survey (24), although the numbers of sampled persons reporting fractures of individual sites are in most instances too small to meet the standards of statistical reliability set by the National Center for Health Statistics. Given this reservation, the bones most often fractured are, in order of frequency, the phalanges of the hand; the tarsal and metatarsal bones; the ribs, sternum, and larynx; the carpal bones; the phalanges of the foot; the radius and ulna; the face bones; the humerus; the clavicle; the tibia and fibula; the vertebral column; the patella; the ankle, and the neck of the femur. Common mechanisms of injuries for fractures of these sites are given in Table 8-5. More details are given by Rockwood and Green (26), Aston (4) and Apley (3). Buhr and Cooke (6) have divided many of the common fractures into four classes, depending both on the etiology and on the sex and age group most frequently affected.

The first class involves such sites as the shaft of the tibia, the clavicle, and the lower end of the humerus. Fractures of these sites usually occur in youth, are generally caused by severe trauma, and have a male-to-female ratio of about 2 to 1. The graphed age distribution of these fractures is L-shaped, with the peak at the young ages. The sex- and age-specific incidence of fractures of the lower end of the humerus seen at a hospital is shown in Figure 8-1.

The second class consists of fractures in bones that are most frequently injured at work, and which consequently tend to occur among people in their wage-earning years. Fractures in the hands and feet are included in this category. These fractures also affect males more frequently than females, although the male-to-female ratio is decreasing with greater participation of females in the work force. Figure 8-2 shows the sex- and age-specific incidence of fractures of the phalanges of the foot seen at the hospital.

Table 8-5 Frequently Occurring Fracture Sites According to Most Common Mechanisms of Injury

Site	Common mechanisms of injury
Distal phalanges of hand	Crush injuries
Proximal and middle phalanges of hand	Direct blows, twisting injuries
Tarsal bones	Falls from heights, hyperextension of foot and ankle
Metatarsal bones	Crush injuries, twisting injuries
Ribs	Direct blows, crush injuries
Sternum	Direct blows, flexion injuries
Carpal bones	Direct blows, falls, twisting injuries
Phalanges of foot	Heavy objects falling on toes
Distal radius	Falls on outstretched hand
Shafts of radius and ulna	Twisting injuries, direct blows, motor vehicle accidents
Face bones	Direct trauma, motor vehicle accidents
Shaft of humerus	Falls on hand or elbow, direct blows, motor vehicle accidents, crush injuries, missile injuries
Neck of humerus	Falls on outstretched hand
Lower end of humerus (elbow)	Falls on outstretched hand (children), falls on elbow (adults), direct blows (adults)
Clavicle	Direct blows, falls on shoulder, falls on outstretched hand
Lateral tibial condyle	Direct blows (especially from automobiles), falls from heights
Shafts of tibia and fibula	Direct blows, twisting injuries, motor vehicle accidents, gunshot wounds, ski injuries, falls
Vertebrae	Crush injuries, direct blows, falls from heights, extension injuries, whiplash injuries, seat-belt injuries, heavy loads on head, gunshot wounds
Patella	Direct blows, falls, sudden contraction of muscles
Ankle	Rotational injuries, falls from heights
Neck of Femur	Falls, twisting injuries

Source: Rockwood and Green (26), Aston (4), Apley (3).

The third class of fractures is often associated with the osteoporotic process, and includes fractures to such sites as the upper end of the femur (the hip), the upper end of the humerus, the vertebrae, and the pelvis. Fractures to these bones are uncommon at younger ages, and are almost always the result of severe trauma when they do occur in young people. The age distribution of these fractures is J-shaped, with a slight peak in

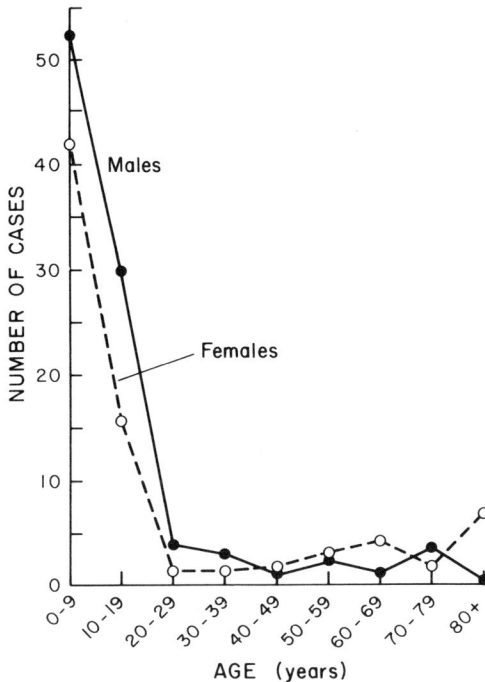

Figure 8-1 Age distribution of cases admitted to a hospital with fracture of the lower end of the humerus.

Source: Buhr and Cooke (6).

youth and a much more marked peak at older ages. At younger ages, these fractures occur more frequently in males than in females, while at older ages they are more common in females than in males. As already mentioned, hip fractures are a particularly important medical problem in older age groups, especially among females. Each year an estimated 2 percent of females and 0.6 percent of males of age 65 years and older will suffer fractured hips (17). The incidence of hip fractures by sex and age is depicted in Figure 8-3.

The final class of fractures contains sites that are most frequently affected in the very young, when bones are still forming, and in the elderly, when osteoporosis is prevalent. Included in this group are fractures occurring in the fibular malleolus (the rounded process on the outside of the ankle), the upper end of the radius, and the lower end of the forearm. In both sexes, the incidence rates are highest in youth and the older ages, but in older ages, females are affected much more frequently than males (2). In Figure 8-4, the sex- and age-specific incidence of fractures of the lower end of the forearm seen in the hospital is shown.

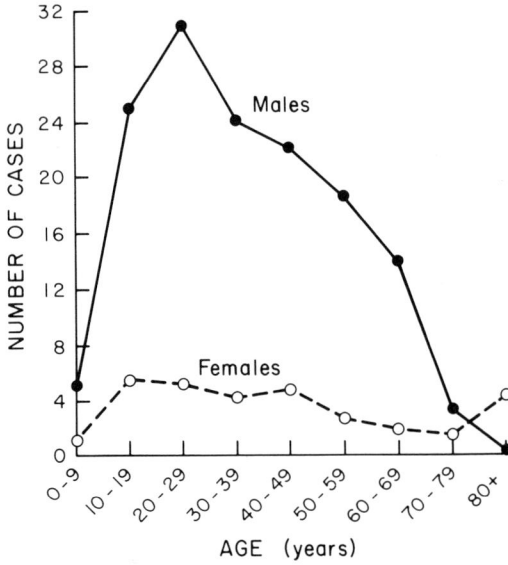

Figure 8-2 Age distribution of cases admitted to a hospital with fracture of the phalanges of the foot.

Source: Buhr and Cooke. (6).

Moderate or severe trauma is clearly a major cause of fractures of all bones during youth and middle age. Severe trauma such as that which may result from automobile accidents, falls from heights, or child-battering accounts for most of the fractures in young children (6,15,20). Sports injuries and highway accidents, such as those in which children on bicycles are struck by motor vehicles, are very common causes of limb fractures in youth (11). Trauma from industrial accidents is a major cause of fractures to people in the wage-earning years. Industrial accidents, in fact, cause 40 percent of all fractures in males of ages 35 to 44 years and 20 percent of fractures in females in this age group (17). Crush injuries and fractures from dropping heavy objects are more common in males than in females, while fractures attributable to stubbing toes occur more frequently in females than males (11).

The proportion of fractures associated with only moderate or minimal trauma rises with increasing age (1,5,6,35,36), although this increase is less marked in males than in females. Considering all ages and types of fractures, about half of the fractures in males but only 1 out of 7 fractures of females are associated with severe trauma. Much of the difference

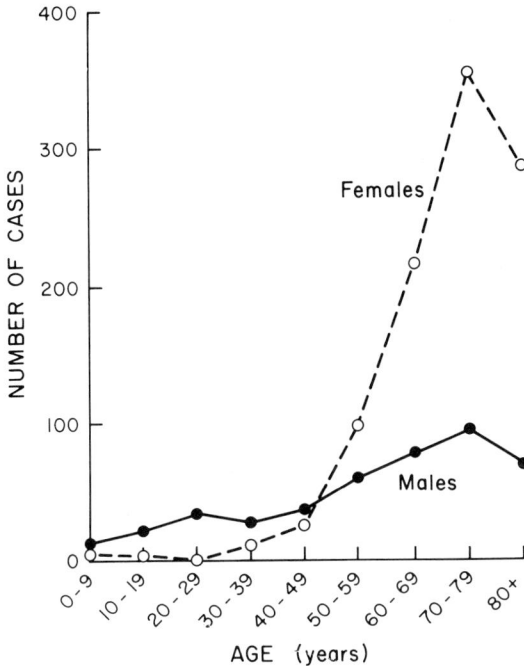

Figure 8-3   Age distribution of cases admitted to a hospital with hip fracture.
Source: Buhr and Cooke (6).

between the sexes is attributable to the large number of fractures associated with only moderate trauma in postmenopausal osteoporotic
women. In people whose bones have become brittle because of an underlying disorder such as osteoporosis, falls are the most common immediate
cause of fracture (5,11,14,16,17,22), but often these falls are associated
with little momentum, such as falls in the course of casual ambulation,
getting out of a chair or bed, or when slipping or tripping. Poor eyesight,
impaired coordination, and diminished muscular strength are additional
predisposing factors for falls and subsequent fractures in the elderly (5).
Transient ischemic attacks may also result in falls and fractures (31,36).
    Osteomalacia, Paget's disease, and primary and secondary tumors in
bone increase the risk for fractures, but these conditions are much less
common than osteoporosis. (The epidemiology of osteoporosis, osteomalacia, and Paget's disease are discussed in Chapter 5, and primary bone
tumors in Chapter 9.) These conditions are sometimes associated with

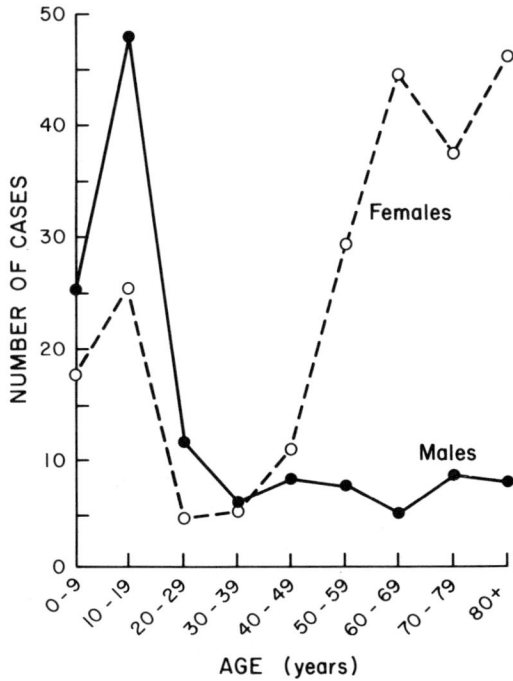

Figure 8-4   Age distribution of cases admitted to a hospital with fracture of the lower end of the forearm.

Source: Buhr and Cooke (6).

pathological fractures, which occur without antecedent trauma in bone that is especially fragile because of an underlying pathological process within the bone. Pathological fractures may occur in a local area of bone destruction, as in the case of neoplasm or Paget's disease, or in a person with weakened bones throughout the skeleton, such as vertebral crush fractures in elderly women with severe osteoporosis. At any age, individuals with osteogenesis imperfecta, a rare condition in which a child is born with bones that are abnormally brittle and susceptible to fracture, are at high risk for pathological fractures.

One final type of fracture that should be mentioned is called fatigue (stress or march) fracture. This type of fracture results from the stress of weight bearing or from antagonistic muscular activity (12,25,32). It occurs most frequently in the second or sometimes the third metatarsal bones of persons with flattened metatarsal arches, so that the heads of the second and third metatarsals are subject to an excessive amount of weight

(4). A fatigue fracture is most likely to occur when ordinarily sedentary people embark on sudden training programs (12), or when there is excessive stress, strain, or muscular activity over a prolonged period, as in military marching and drilling (25,32). At first, the affected person may not be aware of the fatigue fracture and notices only pain and perhaps swelling, but if weight bearing and stressful activity continue, displacement is likely and the fracture becomes obvious (12).

Further research on the epidemiology of fractures could take various directions. Basic descriptive statistics on the frequency of fractures of different sites, including those treated in physicians' offices and on an outpatient basis as well as those seen in hospitals, would be useful. This could probably best be done by combining several years of data from the U.S. Health Interview Survey. Studies designed to identify aspects of the environment which could be modified in order to reduce the likelihood of occurrence of fractures and other injuries would be highly desirable, keeping in mind that the nature of these agents will to a large extent be different for children, young adults, and the elderly. Finally, additional study of factors that influence recovery from fractures of the hip and other sites in the elderly would be important, given the large amount of morbidity and mortality caused by fractures in this age group.

REFERENCES

1. Alffram, P-A. 1964. "An epidemiologic study of cervical and trochanteric fractures of the femur in an urban population." *Acta Orthop. Scand. Suppl.* 65:1–109.
2. ———, and Bauer, G. C. H. 1962. "Epidemiology of fracture of the forearm." *J. Bone Jt. Surg. (Amer.)* 44:105–114.
3. Apley, A. G. 1973, *A System of Orthopaedics and Fractures.* London: Butterworths.
4. Aston, J. N. 1967. *A Short Textbook of Orthopaedics and Traumatology.* Philadelphia: Lippincott.
5. Bauer, G. 1960. "Epidemiology of fracture in aged persons." *Clin. Orthop.* 17:219–225.
6. Buhr, A. J., and Cooke, A. M. 1959. "Fracture patterns." *Lancet* 531–536.
7. Cobey, J. C., Cobey, J. H., Conant, L., Weil, U. H., Greenwald, W. F., and Southwick, W. O. 1976. "Indicators of recovery from fractures of the hip." *Clin. Orthop.* 117:258–262.
8. Duthie, R. D., and Ferguson, A. B., Jr. 1973. *Mercer's Orthopaedic Surgery.* London: Arnold.
9. Eppright, R. H., and Wilkins, K. E. 1975. "Fractures and dislocations of the elbow." In *Fractures.* C. A. Rockwood, Jr. and D. P. Green, eds. Philadelphia: Lippincott, pp. 487–563.
10. Gallannaugh, S. C., Martin, A., and Millard, P. H. 1976. "Regional survey of femoral neck fractures." *Brit Med. J.* 2:1496–1497.

11. Garraway, W. M., Stauffer, R. N., Kurland, L. T., and O'Fallon, W. M. 1979. "Limb fractures in a defined population, frequency and distribution." *Mayo Clinic Proc.* 54:701–707.
12. Graham, C. 1970. "Stress fractures in joggers." *Texas Medicine* 66:68–73.
13. Green, D. P., and Rowland, S. A. 1975. "Fractures and dislocations in the hand." In *Fractures*. C. A. Rockwood, Jr. and D. P. Green, eds. Philadelphia: Lippincott, pp. 265–343.
14. Gyepes, M., Mellins, H. Z., and Katz, I. 1962. "The low incidence of fracture of the hip in the Negro." *J. Amer. Med. Ass.* 181:1073–1074.
15. Heiser, J. M., and Oppenheim, W. 1980. "Fractures of the hip in children. A review of forty cases." *Clin. Orthop.* 149:177–184.
16. Iskrant, A. P. 1968. "The etiology of fractured hips in females." *Amer. J. Pub. Hlth.* 58:485–490.
17. Knowelden, J., Buhr, A. J., and Dunbar, O. 1964. "Incidence of fractures in persons over 35 years of age. A report to the MRC Working Party on fractures in the elderly." *Brit. J. Prev. Soc. Med.* 18:130–141.
18. Kraus, J. F. 1978. "Epidemiologic features of head and spinal cord injury." *Adv. Neurol.* 19:261–278.
19. ———, Franti, C. E., Riggins, R. S., Richards, D., and Borhani, N. O. 1975. "Incidence of traumatic spinal cord lesions." *J. Chron. Dis.* 28:471–492.
20. Lam, S. F. 1971, "Fracture of the neck of the femur in children." *J. Bone Jt. Surg. (Amer.)* 53:1165–1179.
21. Larson, R. L. 1975. "Dislocations and ligamentous injuries of the knee." In *Fractures*. C. A. Rockwood, Jr. and D. P. Green, eds. Philadelphia: Lippincott, pp. 1182–1284.
22. Leitch, I. H., Knowelden, J., and Seddon, H. J. 1964. "Incidence of fractures, particularly of the neck of the femur, in patients in mental hospitals." *Brit. J. Prev. Soc. Med.* 18:142–145.
23. National Center for Health Statistics. 1978. *Acute Conditions. Incidence and Associated Disability,* United States, July 1976–June 1977. DHEW Pub. No. (PHS) 78-1553.
24. ———. 1979. Health Interview Survey, 1975–1976. Unpublished data.
25. Nickerson, S. H. 1943. "March fracture or insufficiency fracture." *Amer. J. Surg.* 62:154–164.
26. Rockwood, C. A., Jr., and Green, D. P. 1975. *Fractures.* Philadelphia: Lippincott.
27. Rowe, C. R. 1956. "Prognosis of dislocations of the shoulder." *J. Bone Jt. Surg. (Amer.)* 38:957–977.
28. ———. 1980. "Acute and recurrent anterior dislocations of the shoulder." *Orthop. Clin. of N. Amer.* 11:253–270.
29. ———, Pierce, D. S., and Clark, J. G. 1973. "Voluntary dislocations of the shoulder." *J. Bone Jt. Surg. (Amer.)* 55:445–460.
30. ———, and Sakellarides, H. T. 1961. "Factors related to recurrences of anterior dislocations of the shoulder." *Clin. Orthop.* 20:40–48.
31. Sheldon, J. H. 1960. "On the natural history of falls in old age." *Brit. Med. J.* 1685–1690.
32. Torisu, T. 1980. "Fatigue fracture of the pelvis after total knee replacements." *Clin. Orthop.* 149:216–219.
33. U.S. Bureau of the Census. 1977. *Current Population Reports, Projection of the Population of the United States, 1977-2050.* Series P-25, No. 704.

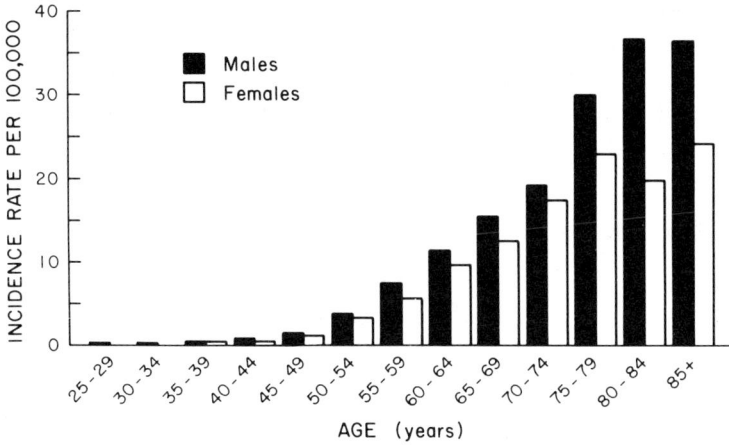

Figure 9-1 Average annual incidence rates per 100,000 for multiple myeloma by age and sex, Connecticut, 1960–1974.

Source: Heston et al. (34).

Little is known of the etiology of multiple myeloma. Trauma was once believed to be an etiologic factor (10,30), but it is likely that trauma simply precipitates noticeable pain in some cases. The possible role of an oncogenic virus in multiple myeloma, which was studied using mouse plasmacytoma as an animal model, has not been substantiated in humans (62). Chromosomal abnormalities, including the translocation known as the Philadelphia chromosome, have been noted in some patients (74), but the significance of this is uncertain.

Environmental factors have received some attention. Although no association between exposure to radiation and multiple myeloma was found during the first twenty years of follow-up of atomic bomb survivors in Hiroshima and Nagasaki, recent data suggest almost a five-fold increase in risk among those exposed to 100 or more rads (36). In Texas (4) it was found that the highest mortality rates for multiple myeloma occurred in areas where relatively high proportions of the population were engaged in farming or were employed in beauty shops or carpentry. Since other data have also suggested higher risks in farmers (52), more detailed study is merited.

The immune system is currently the focus of greatest interest. Impaired immunologic responses associated with multiple myeloma have long been noted (23,30,59,61). Although the bone lesions in multiple myeloma attract attention as the principal site of pain and of abnormal immunoglobulin production, it now appears that bone involvement is only one facet of a generalized defect of the immune system (62). The mechanisms by which normal immune responses break down are thought to be multifactorial (59), but more work is needed to determine the specific processes and underlying etiologic factors.

OSTEOSARCOMA

Osteosarcomas arise from cells concerned with bone formation. In adolescents, osteosarcomas occur most frequently near the growing ends of major long bones, especially the lower femur and the tibia; in older individuals, flat bones such as the ilium are affected most commonly. Metastasis to the lungs and other bones is common, and the prognosis is poor.

Figure 9-2 shows mean annual age-specific incidence rates for selected bone neoplasms in southwestern England from 1946 to 1974, where the annual incidence rate over all ages for osteosarcoma was found to be 2.2 per 1 million for males and 1.9 per 1 million for females (68). Age-specific incidence rates for osteosarcoma are highest during the adolescent and early adult years and to a certain extent again in the older adult years. Somewhat less than half of the cases in the late adult years occur in association with Paget's disease (considered in Chapter 5), probably because of the disturbed osseous metabolism (3,8,14,16,42,44, 50,63,67,68,76). Also, some of the elderly cases may in fact have metastases from other sites and are misclassified as primary osteosarcoma (34).

Among the cases in adolescence and young adulthood, the age of highest incidence occurs earlier for females than for males (19,31,33, 42,46,58), corresponding to the earlier adolescent growth spurt in females. Larsson and Lorentzon (42), for instance, found the peak incidence of osteosarcoma to be 12 years of age for females and 16 years of age for males.

Males are affected more frequently than females by osteosarcoma, with the reported sex ratios for all ages combined ranging from 1.2:1 to 1.5:1 (42,63,68). Among those of ages 15 to 24, however, the male-to-female ratio is almost 2 to 1 (68). Although death rates from osteosarcoma in children appear to be similar in various parts of the United States (31), in Sweden they have been found to be highest in the south, and for all parts of the country, in urban areas (41).

Osteosarcoma in adolescents is almost certainly related in some way to the growth spurt at that time. Acheson (1) has pointed out that anabolic steroid hormones promote accelerated mitosis in all normally growing skeletal tissue, and therefore it is possible that they also stimulate neo-

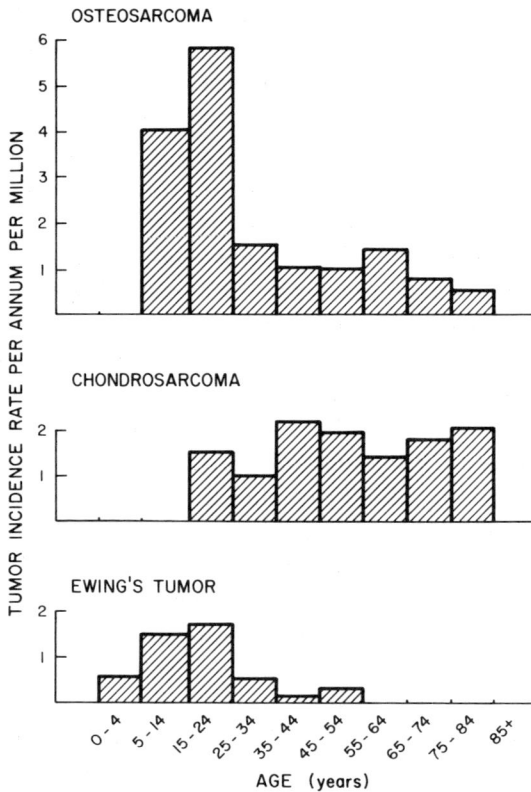

Figure 9-2 Annual incidence rates per 1 million of selected bone neoplasms, by age.

Source: Price and Jeffree (68).

plastic growth in cells with existing malignant potential. On the average, a two- to three-year interval is seen from the time of maximum growth to the peak incidence of bone neoplasms (33) for both males and females. Most of the tumors in adolescents are located at sites of maximal growth, such as the metaphyses of long bones (14,16,58,68,76), suggesting that ossification rather than skeletal enlargement is related to the development of these neoplasms (33). At older ages, the tumor sites are more evenly distributed throughout the skeleton (68,76). The observation that adolescents with osteosarcoma are taller than average has also been cited as evidence that the adolescent growth spurt is in some way related to the onset of at least some osteosarcomas (29).

One established factor for osteosarcoma in adults is exposure to radioactivity. This was first recognized in 1931, when Martland (48) reported an increased risk among watch dial painters who ingested radium when they put brushes with the radioactive radium between their lips. Since then, other groups exposed to sources of radioactivity from within the body, including other radium dial painters (32), radium chemists (20) and those exposed to therapeutic ^{226}Ra (20), have been reported to have on the average a 50-fold increased risk for osteosarcoma (75). Increasing risks have been related to higher doses (25,69), and a shorter average lateney period has been found with higher doses (64). Also, those exposed before the age of about 20 years have considerably higher risks than those exposed at older ages (65). Bones may be especially likely to be affected because radium isotopes result in the formation of radioactive strontium 90, which is in the same chemical family as calcium (63). It appears to be alpha particles that are related specifically to osteosarcoma when the source of exposure to radiation is within the body.

Increased risks may also occur following exposure to external sources of radiation, but so far the evidence is inconclusive. On the one hand, patients with ankylosing spondylitis who have received X-ray treatment appear to have an increased risk estimated to be about 2.5-fold (13). Numerous case reports have noted osteosarcomas associated with external radiation of normal bone, of bone affected with Ewing's tumor, of other organs affected with cancer, and of benign lesions of bone (37,43,71,75). On the other hand, after 20 years of follow-up, data from Hiroshima and Nagasaki survivors did not indicate an increased risk for osteosarcoma among those exposed to nuclear radiation, but it is possible that the period of follow-up was not sufficiently long for an effect to be seen (12).

Some evidence exists that viruses can cause osteosarcoma in animals (25–28). For instance, electron microscopy showed virus-like particles in osteosarcoma in mice who had been injected with an extract of osteosarcomas from another group of mice (28). However, evidence for a viral etiology in humans is lacking (54,55). Neither trauma (50,53) nor heredity (11,14,31) appears to be important etiologically. Finally, the finding that larger breeds of dogs have considerably higher incidence rates of osteosarcoma than smaller breeds (9,72) is of unknown relevance to humans.

OTHER MALIGNANT NEOPLASMS OF BONE

Chondrosarcomas

These tumors, for which the annual incidence rate has been reported as 1.4 per 1 million for males and 1.1 per 1 million for females (68), generally grow much more slowly than osteosarcomas, and are associated with much better survivorship, on the average (21,47). These cartilaginous tumors tend to arise from the ends of the major long bones such as the femur, or from flat bones such as the pelvis, ribs, sternum, and scapula. In Figure 9-2 it may be seen that chondrosarcoma is rare before 15 years of age, but after that age little variation exists in age-specific incidence rates (68). Males are affected more frequently than females in the ratio of 1.2–1.9 to 1 (42,68). At older ages, chondrosarcoma may occur in association with Paget's disease, osteochondroma, or diaphyseal aclasia (the imperfect formation of bone in the cartilage between the diaphysis and epiphysis) (18). Otherwise, etiologic agents for chondrosarcoma are not known.

Ewing's Tumor

Also called Ewing's sarcoma, this tumor usually begins in the marrow at about the middle of the shaft of long bone, but the type of cell from which it originates is not known. The femur, tibia, fibula, and humerus are most frequently affected first, but it tends to spread to the lungs and to other bones throughout the skeleton once it has become established. Ewing's tumor used to be considered almost inevitably fatal in a short period of time, but recently there have been some survivors who were treated with radiotherapy and multiagent chemotherapy (22,24,66,71).

The average annual incidence rate for Ewing's tumor has been reported to be 0.7 per 1 million for males and 0.5 per 1 million for females (68). Figure 9-2 showed that the age distribution is in general similar to that for osteosarcoma. Some reports show the peak age during adolescence to be similar for males and females (42), while others have found an earlier peak in females than in males (31,66). Ewing's tumor affects males about twice as frequently as females (6,15,24,40,42,66). Particularly high mortality rates for males, but low rates for females, have been reported in New England (31). Ewing's tumor has been found more frequently in the southeast of Sweden than elsewhere in that country, but, unlike osteosarcoma, there is no urban-rural gradient (40). Its etiology is unknown.

REFERENCES

1. Acheson, R. M. 1963. "A hypothesis regarding the possible role of anabolic steroid hormones as promotors of neoplasia of bone and bone marrow at adolescence." *Yale J. Biol. Med.* 36:43–52.

2. Advani, S. H., Soman, C. S., Talwalkar, G. V., Iyer, Y. S., and Bhatia, H. M. 1978. "Multiple myeloma: Review of 231 cases." *Indian J. Cancer* 15:55–61.
3. Aegerter, E., and Kirkpatrick, J. A., Jr. 1975. *Orthopedic Diseases.* Philadelphia: Saunders.
4. Agu, V. U., Christensen, B. L., and Buffler, P. A. 1980. "Geographic patterns of multiple myeloma: racial and industrial correlates, state of Texas, 1969–71." *J. Natl. Canc. Inst.* 65:735–738.
5. Best, W. R., Pisciotta, A. V., Donnelly, W. J., Fowler, W. M., Linman, J. W., Schwartz, S. O., and Louis, J. 1963. "Diagnosis and course of multiple myeloma, with survival estimations." *J. Lab. Clin. Med.* 62:860.
6. Bhansali, S. K., and Desai, P. B. 1963. "Ewing's sarcoma. Observations on 107 cases." *J. Bone Jt. Surg. (Amer.)* 45:541–553.
7. Blattner, W. A., Jacobson, R. J., and Shulman, G. 1979. "Multiple myeloma in South African blacks." (letter) *Lancet* 1:928–929.
8. Boyd, J. T., Doll, R., Hill, G. B., and Sissons, H. A. 1969. "Mortality from primary tumors of bone in England and Wales 1961–63." *Brit. J. Prev. Soc. Med.* 23:12–22.
9. Brodey, R. S., and Riser, W. H. 1969. "Canine osteosarcoma. A clinico-pathologic study of 194 cases." *Clin. Orthop.* 62:54–64.
10. Coley, W. B., and Coley, B. L. 1926. "Primary malignant tumors of the long bones; end-results in one hundred and seventy operable cases." *Arch. Surg.* 13:779–836, 14:63–141.
11. Colyer, R. A. 1979. "Osteogenic sarcoma in siblings." *Johns Hopkins Med. J.* 145:131–135.
12. Committee on the Biological Effects of Ionizing Radiation (BEIR Committee). 1980. *The Effects on Populations of Exposure to Low Levels of Ionizing Radiation: 1980.* Washington: National Academy Press.
13. Court Brown, W. M., and Doll, R. 1965. "Mortality from cancer and other causes after radiotherapy for ankylosing spondylitis." *Brit. Med. J.* 2:1327–1332.
14. Dahlin, D. C. 1978. *Bone Tumors. General Aspects and Data on 6221 Cases.* Springfield, Ill.: Charles C Thomas.
15. ———. Coventry, M. B., and Scanlon, P. W. 1961. "Ewing's sarcoma: A critical analysis of 165 cases." *J. Bone Jt. Surg. (Amer.)* 43:185–192.
16. ———, and Coventry, M. B. 1967. "Osteogenic sarcomas. A study of 600 cases." *J. Bone Jt. Surg. (Amer.)* 49:101–110.
17. Dawson, A. A., and Ogston, D. 1973. "High incidence of myelomatosis in northeast Scotland." *Scottish Med. J.* 18:75–77.
18. Duthie, R. B., and Ferguson, A. B., Jr. 1973. *Mercer's Orthopaedic Surgery.* London: Arnold.
19. Ederer, F., Miller, R. W., and Scotto, J. 1965. "U.S. childhood cancer mortality patterns, 1950–1959. Etiologic implications." *J. Amer. Med. Ass.* 192:593–596.
20. Evans, R. D. 1966. "The effects of skeletally deposited alpha-ray emitters in man." *Brit. J. Radiol.* 39:881–895.
21. Evans, H. L., Ayala, A. G., and Romsdahl, M. M. 1977. "Prognostic factors in chondrosarcoma of bone." *Cancer* 40:818–831.
22. Evarts, C. M., and Rubin, P. 1978. "Bone tumors." In *Clinical Oncology for Medical Students and Physicians.* P. Rubin and R. F. Bakemeier, eds. Rochester, N.Y.: American Cancer Society, pp. 203–207.
23. Fahey, J. L., Scoggins, R., Utz, J. P., and Szwed, C. 1963. "Infection, antibody response and gamma globulin components in multiple myeloma, and macroglobulinemia." *Amer. J. Med.* 35:698–707.

24. Fernandez, C. M., Lindberg, R. D., Sutlow, W. W., and Samuels, M. L. 1974. "Localized Ewing's Sarcoma—Treatment and end results." *Cancer* 34:143–148.
25. Finkel, M. P., and Biskis, B. O. 1968. "Experimental induction of osteosarcomas." *Progr. Exp. Tumor Res.* 10:72–111.
26. ———, Biskis, B. O., and Farrell, C. 1968. "Osteosarcomas appearing in Syrian hamsters after treatment with extracts of human osteosarcomas." *Proc. Natl. Acad. Sci.* 60:1223–1230.
27. ——— et al. 1969. "Nonmalignant and malignant changes in hamsters inoculated with extracts of human osteosarcomas." *Radiology* 92:1546–1552.
28. ———, Biskis, B. O., and Jinkins, P. B. 1966. "Virus induction of osteosarcoma in mice." *Science* 151:698–700.
29. Fraumeni, J. F., Jr. 1966. "Stature and malignant tumors of bone in childhood and adolescence." *Cancer* 20:967–973.
30. Geschickter, C. F., and Copeland, M. M. 1928. "Multiple myeloma." *Arch. Surg.* 16:807–863.
31. Glass, A. G., and Fraumeni, J. F. 1970. "Epidemiology of bone cancer in children." *J. Natl. Cancer Inst.* 44:187–199.
32. Hasterlik, R. J., Finkel, A. J., and Miller, L. E. 1964. "The cancer hazards of industrial and accidental exposure to radioactive isotopes." *Ann. N.Y. Acad. Sci.* 114:832–837.
33. Hems, G. 1970. "Aetiology of bone cancer, and some other cancers, in the young." *Brit. J. Cancer* 24:202–214.
34. Heston, J. F., Kelly, J. B., Meigs, J. W., Flannery, J. T., Honeyman, M. S., and Lloyd, D. S. 1981. *Forty Years of Cancer in Connecticut: 1935–1974.* Cancer in Connecticut Monograph Series 1980–1. In press.
35. Innes, J., and Newall, J. 1961. "Myelomatosis." *Lancet* 1:239–245.
36. Ishimaru, T. 1979. "More on radiation exposure and multiple myeloma." (letter) *New Engl. J. Med.* 301:439–440.
37. Kim, J. H., Chu, F. C., Woodard, H. Q., Melamed, M. R., Huvos, A., and Cantin, J. 1978. "Radiation-induced soft-tissue and bone sarcoma." *Radiology* 129:501–508.
38. Kyle, R. A. 1975. "Multiple myeloma: Review of 869 cases." *Mayo Clin. Proc.* 50:29–40.
39. ———, Nobrega, F. T., and Kurland, L. T. 1969. "Multiple myeloma in Olmsted County, Minnesota, 1945–1964." *Blood* 33:739–745.
40. Larsson, S. E., Boquist, L., and Bergdahl, L. 1973. "Ewing's sarcoma. A consecutive series of 64 cases diagnosed in Sweden 1958–1967." *Clin. Orthop.* 95:263–272.
41. ———, and Lorentzon, R. 1974. "The geographic variation of incidence of malignant primary bone tumors in Sweden." *J. Bone Jt. Surg. (Amer.)* 56:592–600.
42. Larsson, S. E., and Lorentzon, R. 1974. "The incidence of malignant primary bone tumors in relation to age, sex, and site." *J. Bone Jt. Surg. (Brit.)* 56:534–540.
43. Lewis, R. J., Marcove, R. C., Rosen, G. 1977. "Ewing's sarcoma—Functional effects of radiation therapy." *J. Bone Jt. Surg. (Amer.)* 59:325–331.
44. Mackenzie, A., Court Brown, W. M., Doll, R., and Sissons, H. A. 1961. "Mortality from primary tumors of bone in England and Wales." *Brit. Med. J.* 1:1782–1790.
45. MacMahon, B., and Clark, D. W. 1956. "The incidence of multiple myeloma." *J. Chron. Dis.* 4:508–515.
46. Marcove, R. C., Miké, V., Hajck, J. V., Levin, A. G., and Hutter, R. V. P. 1970.

"Osteogenic sarcoma under the age of twenty-one. A review of one hundred and forty-five operative cases." *J. Bone Jt. Surg. (Amer.)* 52:411–423.

47. ———. Miké V., Hutter, R. V. P., Huvos, A. G., Shoji, H., Miller, T. R., and Kosloff, R. 1972. "Chondrosarcoma of the pelvis and upper end of the femur." *J. Bone Jt. Surg. (Amer.)* 54:561–572.

48. Martland, H. S. 1931. "The occurrence of malignancy in radioactive persons." *Amer. J. Cancer* 15:2435–2516.

49. McFarlane, H. 1966. "Multiple myeloma in Jamaica: A study of 40 cases with special reference to the incidence and laboratory diagnosis." *J. Clin. Path.* 19:268–271.

50. McKenna, R. J., Schwinn, C. P., Soong, K. Y., and Higinbotham, N. L. 1966. "Sarcomata of the osteogenic series (osteosarcoma, fibrosarcoma, chondrosarcoma, parosteal osteogenic sarcoma, and sarcomata arising in abnormal bone). An analysis of 552 cases." *J. Bone Jt. Surg. (Amer.)* 48:1–25.

51. McPhedran, P. 1972. "Multiple myeloma incidence in metropolitan Atlanta, Georgia: Rural and seasonal variation." *Blood* 39:866–873.

52. Milham, S., Jr. 1971. "Leukemia and multiple myeloma in farmers." *Amer. J. Epid.* 94:307–310.

53. Monkman, G. R., Orwoll, G., and Ivins, J. C. 1974. "Trauma and oncogenesis." *Mayo Clinic Proc.* 49:157–163.

54. Moore, M. 1971. "Tumour-specific antigens: Their possible significance in the etiology and treatment of malignant disease." *J. Bone Jt. Surg. (Brit.)* 53:13–22.

55. Morton, D. L., and Malmgren, R. A. 1968. "Human osteosarcomas: Immunologic evidence suggesting an associated infectious agent." *Science* 162:1279–1281.

56. National Center for Health Statistics. 1980. *Vital Statistics of the United States, 1976. Volume II—Mortality.* Washington, U.S. Government Printing Office. DHHS Publication No. (PHS) 80–1101.

57. Nauts, H. C. 1975. *Multiple Myeloma: Beneficial Effects of Acute Infections or Immunotherapy* (Bacterial Vaccines). Monograph #13, Cancer Research Institute, New York, N.Y.

58. Ohno, T., Abe, M., Tateishi, A., Kako, K., Miki, H., Sekine, K., Ueyama, H., Hasegawa, O., and Obara, K. 1975. "Osteogenic sarcoma. A study of one hundred and thirty cases." *J. Bone Jt. Surg (Amer.)* 57:397–404.

59. Paglieroni, T., and MacKenzie, M. R. 1977. "Studies on the pathogenesis of an immune defect in multiple myeloma." *J. Clin. Invest.* 59:1120–1133.

60. ———, MacKenzie, M. R., and Caggiano, V. 1978. "Multiple myeloma: An immunologic profile. II. Bone marrow studies." *J. Natl. Canc. Inst.* 61:943–950.

61. Paredes, J. M., and Mitchell, B. S. 1980. "Multiple myeloma: Current concepts in diagnosis and management." *Med. Clin. N. Am.* 64:729–742.

62. Parker, D., and Malpas, J. S. 1979. "Multiple myeloma." *J. Roy. Coll. Phys. London* 13:146–153.

63. Phillips, A. J. 1965. "A mortality study of primary tumors of bone in Canada." *Can. Med. Assoc. J.* 92:391–393.

64. Polednak, A. P. 1978. "Bone cancer among female radium dial workers. Latency periods and incidence rates by time after exposure: Brief communication." *J. Natl. Cancer Inst.* 60:77–82.

65. ———, Stehney, A. F., and Rowland, R. E. 1978. "Mortality among women first employed before 1930 in the U.S. radium dial-painting industry." *Amer. J. Epid.* 107:179–195.

66. Pomeroy, T. C., and Johnson, R. E. 1975. "Prognostic factors for survival in Ewing's sarcoma." *Amer. J. Roent.* 123:598–606.

67. Price, C. H. G. 1958. "Primary bone-forming tumours and their relationship to skeletal growth." *J. Bone Jt. Surg. (Brit.)* 40:574–593.

68. ———, and Jeffree, G. M. 1977. "Incidence of bone sarcoma in S.W. England, 1946–74, in relation to age, sex, tumour site, and histology." *Brit. J. Cancer* 36:511–522.

69. Rowland, R. E., Stehney, A. F., and Lucas, H. F., Jr. 1978. "Dose-response relationship for female radium dial workers." *Radiation Res.* 76:368–383.

70. Stober, J., and Asal, N. R. 1976. "Multiple myeloma in Oklahoma: Racial, age, sex, geographic and time variations." *Southern Med. J.* 69:298–302.

71. Strong, L. C., Herson, J., Osborne, B. M., and Sutlow, W. W. 1979. "Risk of radiation-related subsequent malignant tumors in survivors of Ewing's sarcoma." *J. Natl. Cancer Inst.* 62:1401–1406.

72. Tjalma, R. A. 1966. "Canine bone sarcoma: Estimation of relative risk as a function of body size." *J. Nat. Cancer Inst.* 36:1137–1150.

73. Tozer, R. A., Clear, A. S., Davies, D. R., and Hutt, M. S. R. 1980. "Unusual presentation of patients with myelomatosis in Malawi." *J. Clin. Pathol.* 33:544–546.

74. Van Den Berghe, H., Louwagie, A., Broeckaert-Van Orshoven, A., David, G., Virwilghen, R., Michaux, J. L., and Sokal, G. 1979. "Philadelphia chromosome in human multiple myeloma." *J. Natl. Canc. Inst.* 63:11–16.

75. Vaughan, J. M. 1973. *The Effects of Irradiation on the Skeleton.* Glasgow: Oxford University Press.

76. Weinfeld, M. S., and Dudley, H. R. 1962. "Osteogenic sarcoma: A follow-up study of the ninety-four cases observed at the Massachusetts General Hospital from 1920 to 1960." *J. Bone Jt. Surg. (Amer.)* 44:269–276.

Index

34. Wilson, F. C. 1975. "Fractures and dislocations of the ankle." In *Fractures*. C. A. Rockwood, Jr. and D. P. Green, eds. Philadelphia: Lippincott, pp. 1361–1399.
35. Wong, P. C. 1966. "Fracture epidemiology in a mixed Southeastern Asian community (Singapore)." *Clin. Orthop.* 45:55–61.
36. ———. 1967. "Prevention of femoral neck fractures in the elderly." *Geriatrics* 156–163.

9 Bone Neoplasms

Primary neoplasms of bone are not common, but they are, nevertheless, the fourth-leading cause of death among cancers in children (56). Sixty to 75 percent of bone neoplasms are malignant, and the presenting symptom is usually pain (14,22,50,58). Table 9-1 shows an adaptation of a classification scheme of Evarts and Rubin (22) for bone tumors. It may be seen that malignant neoplasms can arise from bone-forming tissue, bone digesting tissue, cartilage, fibrous tissue, marrow, and vascular tissue. Metastatic neoplasms from cancers elsewhere in the body are common, but will not be considered here.

Multiple myeloma is the most frequent type, followed by osteosarcoma, then chondrosarcoma and Ewing's tumor (14,22). Benign neoplasms will not be discussed here except to mention that 40 percent are osteochondroma, a neoplasm that affects males one and a half times more frequently than females and that is seen primarily in persons below the age of 20 years (14). For a detailed description of all bone neoplasms, the reader is referred to Dahlin (14).

Because of the relative rarity of these malignant neoplasms, data on osteosarcoma, chondrosarcoma, Ewing's tumor, and other still less frequently occurring neoplasms of bone, joints, and articular cartilage (ICD 170.0–170.9) are often combined. The Connecticut Tumor Registry (34) reports that annual age-adjusted incidence rates for these malignant neoplasms of bones, joints, and articular cartilage were 0.76 per 100,000 in males and 0.51 per 100,000 in females from 1970 to 1974. Multiple myeloma, which is classified separately, had age-adjusted incidence rates of

Table 9-1   Classification of Malignant Neoplasms of Bone by Origin and Cell Type

Type of neoplasm	Origin	Cell type

Osteosarcoma
  Medullary
  Parosteal
	Bone forming	Osteoblast
		  (forms osteoid)

Osteoclastoma
  (giant cell tumor)
	Bone digesting	Osteoclast
		  (forms no matrix)

Chondrosarcoma
  Primary
  Secondary
	Cartilage	Chondroblast
		  (forms cartilage
		  matrix)

Fibrosarcoma	Fibrous	Fibroblast (forms collagen)
Multiple myeloma Reticulum cell sarcoma	Marrow	Reticuloendothelial system
Angiosarcoma	Vascular	Blood vessel
Adamantinoma of long bones	Uncertain	Uncertain
Ewing's tumor	Uncertain	Uncertain
Spindle cell sarcoma	Uncertain	Uncertain

Source: Evarts and Rubin (22).

3.7 per 100,000 in males and 3.0 per 100,000 in females over this same time period in Connecticut (34).

MULTIPLE MYELOMA

Multiple myeloma (also called plasmacytic myeloma, plasma cell myeloma, myelomatosis, and Kahler's disease) is a malignant disease of plasma cells that typically involves the bone marrow of flat bones, but may affect other tissues as well. The ribs, sternum, clavicle, vertebrae, skull, and pelvis, and also the upper ends of the femur and humerus are most frequently affected. The basic pathologic process is now believed to be the neoplastic proliferation of a single clone of plasma cells that produce a specific protein as if under continual antigenic stimulation. The protein, or "m component," is a monoclonal immunoglobulin molecule or light-chain fragment that frequently can be found in the serum or urine of patients with multiple myeloma (2,38,60,61).

Severe localized pain in bone is usually the first symptom. This pain occurs most often in the back or chest, but occasionally starts in the extremities. Severe anemia, renal insufficiency, and infection are also common. As the disease progresses, many bones are usually affected, and a variety of other local and systemic symptoms are seen. Pathologic fractures may occur, and spinal involvement may result in marked postural changes, pain in nerve roots, and occasionally paraplegia. X-rays usually reveal multiple "punched out" areas of the bone destruction. The diagnostic criteria commonly used for multiple myeloma include (1) increasing numbers of abnormal, atypical, or immature plasma cells in the bone marrow, or histologic evidence of plasmacytoma, (2) the presence of monoclonal protein in serum or urine, and (3) X-ray evidence of bone lesions consistent with those of myeloma (38). The disease is uniformly fatal, although there is some variation in length of survival.

Reported incidence rates for multiple myeloma in the United States, England, Scotland, and Sweden range from about 1.0 to 3.5 per 100,000 (17,34,39,45). In several areas, incidence rates and mortality rates have been increasing over the past few decades (34,38,45,70), but this may be attributable to improved diagnosis and increased use of medical care.

The vast majority of cases occur in people over 50 years of age (2,5,30,34,38,39,57,70). Within this range, the age group with the highest incidence has differed from one study to another, but population-based studies generally show greater incidence rates with increasing age (Figure 9-1) (34,38). Also, males are affected somewhat more often than females, with the reported male-to-female ratios ranging between 1.3 to 1 and 2 to 1 (2,5,7,17,30,34,35,39,45,49,57,70).

Studies in the United States, Malawi, South Africa, and Jamaica have indicated that incidence rates are higher in blacks than in whites (45,49,51,62,70,73). MacMahon and Clark (45), for instance, reported age-standardized mean annual incidence rates of 2.5 per 100,000 among blacks and 1.0 per 100,000 among whites in Brooklyn during the years from 1943 to 1952. In a South African study (7) age-adjusted incidence rates of 7.5 per 100,000 in black males and 5.1 per 100,000 in black females were found. Since failure to identify cases would be expected to be more common among blacks than whites, it is felt that the higher risk in blacks is real (7). One other observation on racial differences was reported from San Francisco, where relatively high rates were found in elderly blacks, but particularly low rates in Chinese (62).

TELEPEN

9036931 9